Parent's Guide to
CHILDHOOD
IMMUNIZATIONS

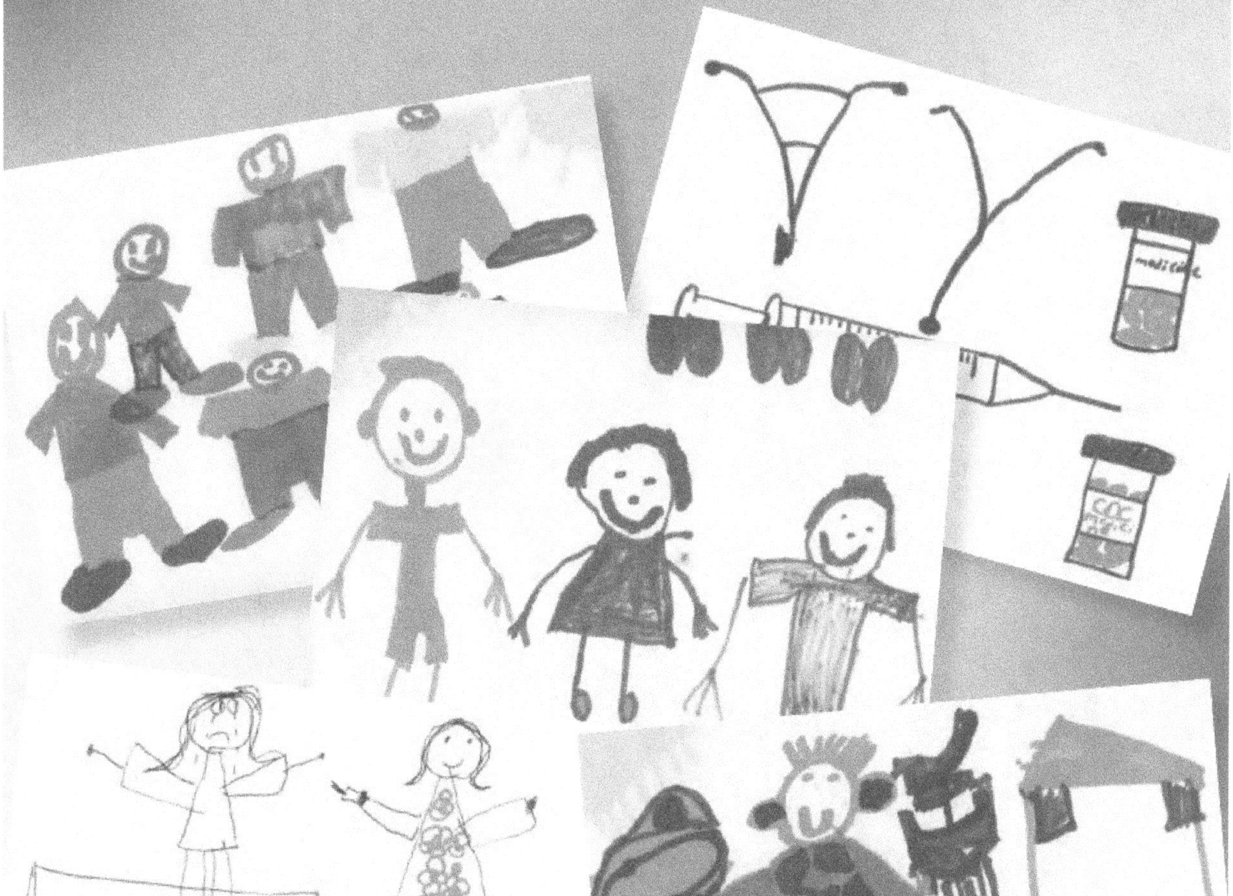

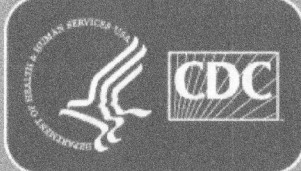

**U.S. Department of
Health and Human Services**
Centers for Disease
Control and Prevention

In 1796, Edward Jenner inoculated an 8-year-old boy against smallpox and coined the term "vaccination" to describe what he had done. Today, smallpox is a memory thanks to vaccination, and routine vaccination against childhood diseases is an important part of our children's health care.

As parents we want to do everything we can to keep our babies from getting sick. In this booklet you will learn more about the role vaccines play in keeping them healthy. You will learn about:

- Diseases that are prevented by vaccines, and the vaccines that prevent them.

- How to prepare for a doctor's visit that includes vaccinations, and what to expect during and after the visit.

- How vaccines help your baby's immune system do its job.

- What is in vaccines, how well they work, and how safe they are.

- Where to find more information.

Table of Contents

2nd Reprint 03/12

Table of Contents

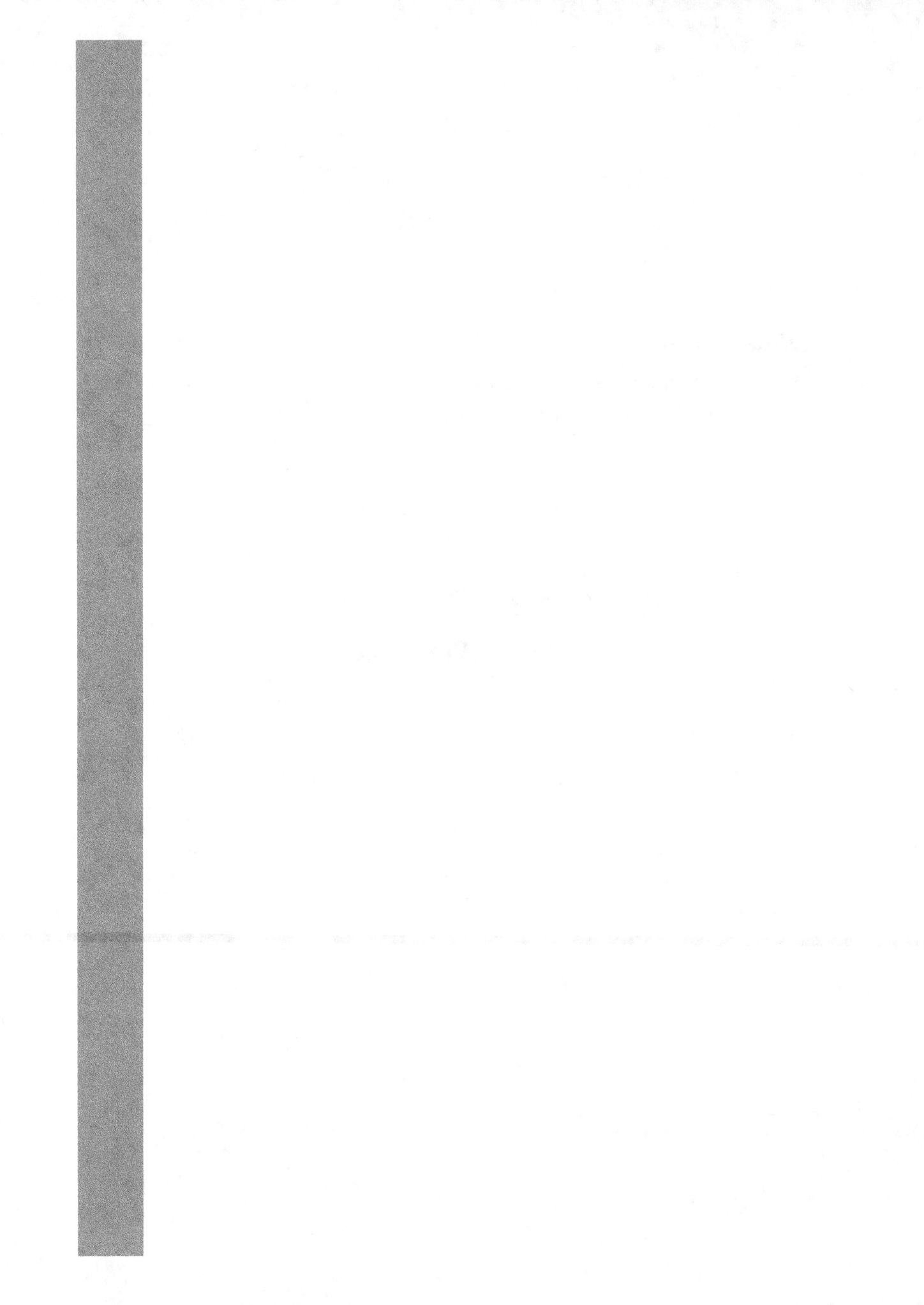

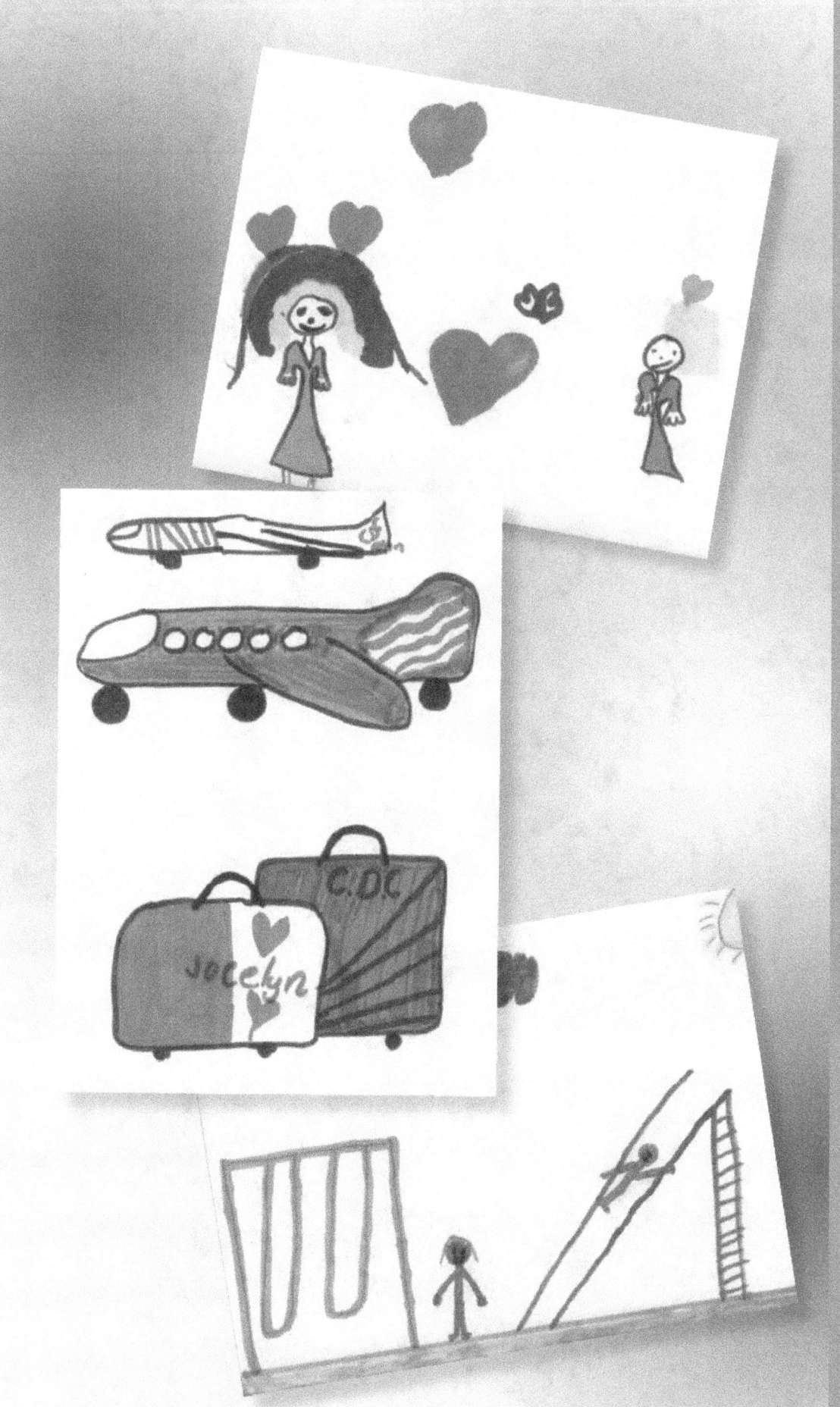

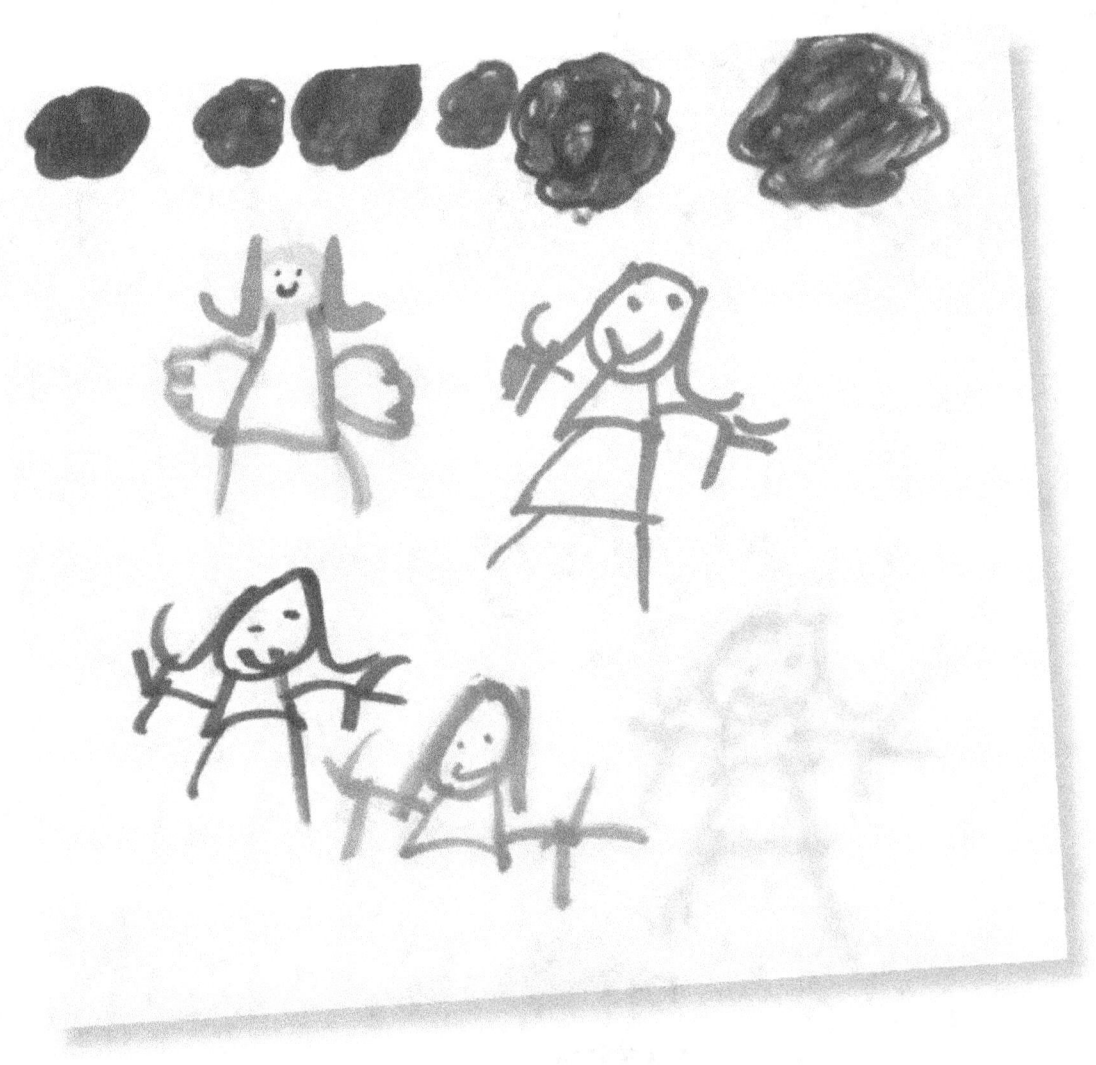

Part 1: Vaccine-Preventable Diseases and Childhood Vaccines

Diseases

Here are the 14 diseases that can be prevented with routine childhood vaccination, and a brief description of each disease:

Diphtheria
Hepatitis A
Hepatitis B
Hib
Influenza (flu)
Measles

Mumps
Pertussis
(whooping cough)
Pneumococcal Disease
Polio
Rotavirus

Rubella
Tetanus
Varicella
(chickenpox)

Diphtheria

Diphtheria is caused by bacteria that live in the mouth and throat of an infected person and cause a sore throat, fever and chills. If diptheria is not properly diagnosed and treated, the bacteria can produce a toxin that causes serious complications such as heart failure and paralysis. About one person in 10 dies. Diphtheria used to be a major cause of childhood illness and death. It is spread from person to person through sneezing, coughing, or even breathing. Through the 1920s about 150,000 people a year got diphtheria, and about 15,000 of them died.

Hepatitis A

Hepatitis A virus causes liver disease, which can result in fever, loss of appetite, fatigue, stomach pain, vomiting, and yellow skin or eyes (jaundice). Children younger than about 6 years old might not show any symptoms. About 100 people die each year from liver failure caused by hepatitis A. Hepatitis A virus is found mainly in bowel movements, and is spread by personal contact or through contaminated food or water.

Hepatitis B

Hepatitis B virus also causes liver disease (the word hepatitis comes from the Greek words for "liver" and "inflammation"). It is spread through contact with blood and other body fluids. Hepatitis B infection can cause muscle or stomach pains, diarrhea or vomiting, yellow skin or eyes (jaundice) or loss of appetite and fatigue. People usually recover after several weeks, but some of them become "chronically infected." These people can spread the disease to others through unprotected sex, sharing needles, or other exposures to blood. Chronically infected people often suffer from cirrhosis (scarring of the liver) or liver cancer, and about 3,000 to 5,000 die each year. Health care workers are at increased risk, as are police officers and other public service workers. A mother who is chronically infected with hepatitis B virus is very likely to infect her baby at birth. Other than babies of infected mothers, children aren't at particularly high risk. But vaccinating children is a practical way to insure that they will be protected later in life when they could be at risk. Rates of hepatitis B have dropped significantly since we began vaccinating children in 1991.

Haemophilus influenzae type b (Hib)

Before there was a vaccine for it, Hib disease was the leading cause of bacterial meningitis in children younger than 5. As recently as the mid-1980s it struck one child out of every 200 in that age group. About 1 in 4 of these children suffered permanent brain damage, and about 1 in 20 died. Hib bacteria are spread through the air by coughing, sneezing and breathing. If they enter the bloodstream, they can cause meningitis, pneumonia, inflammation of the throat, arthritis, and other problems.

Influenza (Flu)

Flu is a seasonal illness, occurring mainly during the winter. It causes fever, sore throat, cough, headache, chills and muscle aches, and can lead to sinus infections, pneumonia, inflammation of the heart, and death. Flu causes more deaths each year than any other vaccine-preventable disease. Most of these deaths are among the elderly, but flu also kills children. Hospitalization rates are high among children, especially those under 1 year old.

Measles

Measles virus causes a rash all over the body, fever, runny nose and cough. About 1 child in 10 also gets an ear infection, up to 1 in 20 gets pneumonia, 1 in 1,000 gets encephalitis, and 1 or 2 in 1,000 die. Before there was a vaccine nearly every child in the United States got measles by age 15. About 450 died each year, 48,000 were hospitalized, 7,000 had seizures, and about 1,000 suffered permanent brain damage. Measles still kills about a half million people a year around the world. Measles is extremely contagious, and is spread through the air by coughing, sneezing, and even breathing.

Vaccine Trivia:

The word "measles" probably comes from a Latin word meaning "miserable."

In 1970, astronaut Ken Mattingly could not participate in the Apollo XIII moon mission because he had been exposed to measles.

Mumps

Mumps is a relatively mild disease, causing fever, headache, and inflammation of the salivary glands, which causes swelling of the cheeks and jaws. It can lead to meningitis in about 1 child in 10, and occasionally to encephalitis or deafness (about 1 in 20,000) or death (about 1 in 10,000). It is spread from person to person through the air. It used to be a very common childhood disease.

Pertussis (Whooping Cough)

Pertussis is caused by a bacteria. It can look like a common cold at first, but after 1 or 2 weeks a child with pertussis is overcome with coughing spells so violent that they interfere with eating, drinking, and even breathing. Pertussis can lead to pneumonia, seizures, encephalopathy (brain infection), and death. Like most childhood vaccine-preventable diseases, pertussis is spread through the air from person to person. Pertussis rates have been increasing in recent years, with more than half of cases occuring among children who are not completely immunized.

Pneumococcal Disease

After Hib disease began to decline, thanks to Hib vaccine, pneumococcal disease became the most common cause of bacterial meningitis in children under 5. Caused by a bacteria and spread through the air, pneumococcal disease also causes ear infections, blood infections, and death. It is most common in winter and early spring. Some groups, including African Americans, some Native American tribes, children with sickle cell disease or HIV nfection, and children without a functioning spleen, are at increased risk for pneumococcal disease.

Polio

Anyone old enough to remember the 1950s will remember the panic caused by polio – a virus that left up to 20,000 people paralyzed each year, unable to walk or sometimes even to breathe. About 1,200 people in the United States were permanently confined to 700-pound "iron lungs" to enable them to breathe, and about 20 of these polio victims still live in them today. Thanks to polio vaccine, there has not been a case of polio in the United States in years.

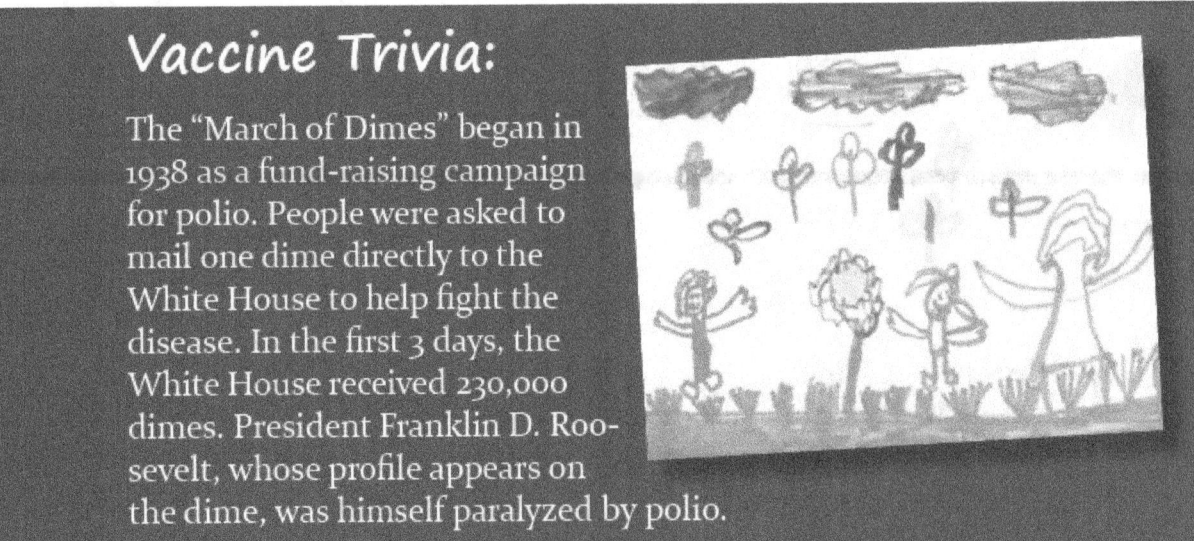

Vaccine Trivia:

The "March of Dimes" began in 1938 as a fund-raising campaign for polio. People were asked to mail one dime directly to the White House to help fight the disease. In the first 3 days, the White House received 230,000 dimes. President Franklin D. Roosevelt, whose profile appears on the dime, was himself paralyzed by polio.

Rotavirus

Rotavirus causes gastroenteritis (diarrhea and vomiting) in young children. Before vaccines, rotavirus infection was responsible for more than 400,000 physician visits, 200,000 emergency department visits, up to 70,000 hospitalizations, and 20 to 60 deaths a year, and cost about a billion dollars a year in time lost from work to care for sick children.

Rubella (German Measles)

Rubella is generally a mild disease, caused by the rubella virus. It causes swollen glands in the back of the neck, a slight fever, rash on the face and neck, and sometimes arthritis-like symptoms in the joints. It is usually spread through the air. However, the greatest danger from rubella is to unborn babies. If a woman gets rubella early in her pregnancy, there is an 80% chance her baby will be born deaf or blind, with a damaged heart or small brain, or mentally impaired. This is called Congenital Rubella Syndrome, or CRS. Miscarriages are also common among women who are infected with rubella during pregnancy. In 1964-65, before there was a vaccine, a major rubella epidemic in the United States infected 12.5 million people and led to 20,000 cases of CRS.

Tetanus (Lockjaw)

Tetanus is different from other vaccine-preventable diseases in that it does not spread from person to person. Children (and adults) become infected when the bacteria enter through breaks in the skin – usually cuts or puncture wounds. About 3 weeks after exposure, a child might get a headache, become cranky, and have spasms in the jaw muscles. The bacteria can then produce a toxin that spreads through the body causing painful muscle cramps in the neck, arms, legs, and stomach. These can be strong enough to break a child's bones, and a child might have to spend several weeks in the hospital under intensive care. About 2 people out 10 who develop tetanus die.

Varicella (Chickenpox)

Before vaccine, almost every child in the United States (about 4 million each year) got chickenpox. The main symptom of chickenpox is an itchy rash all over the body, usually along with fever and drowsiness. It spreads from person to person through the air, or through contact with fluid from the rash. Chickenpox is usually mild, but it can cause skin infections and encephalitis. Among infants less than a year old who get chickenpox, about 4 in 100,000 die. A pregnant woman who gets chickenpox around the time of delivery can infect her baby, and about 1 in 3 of these babies will die if not treated quickly. After a person recovers from chickenpox, the virus stays in the body and can re-emerge years later to cause a painful condition called shingles.

Notice that a common theme in these descriptions is how harmful or prevalent these diseases used to be. Today, a pediatrician might practice for many years and never see a single case of measles, or pertussis, or Hib. Why? Because most parents make sure their children are vaccinated against childhood diseases, and this has resulted in a dramatic decline in disease.

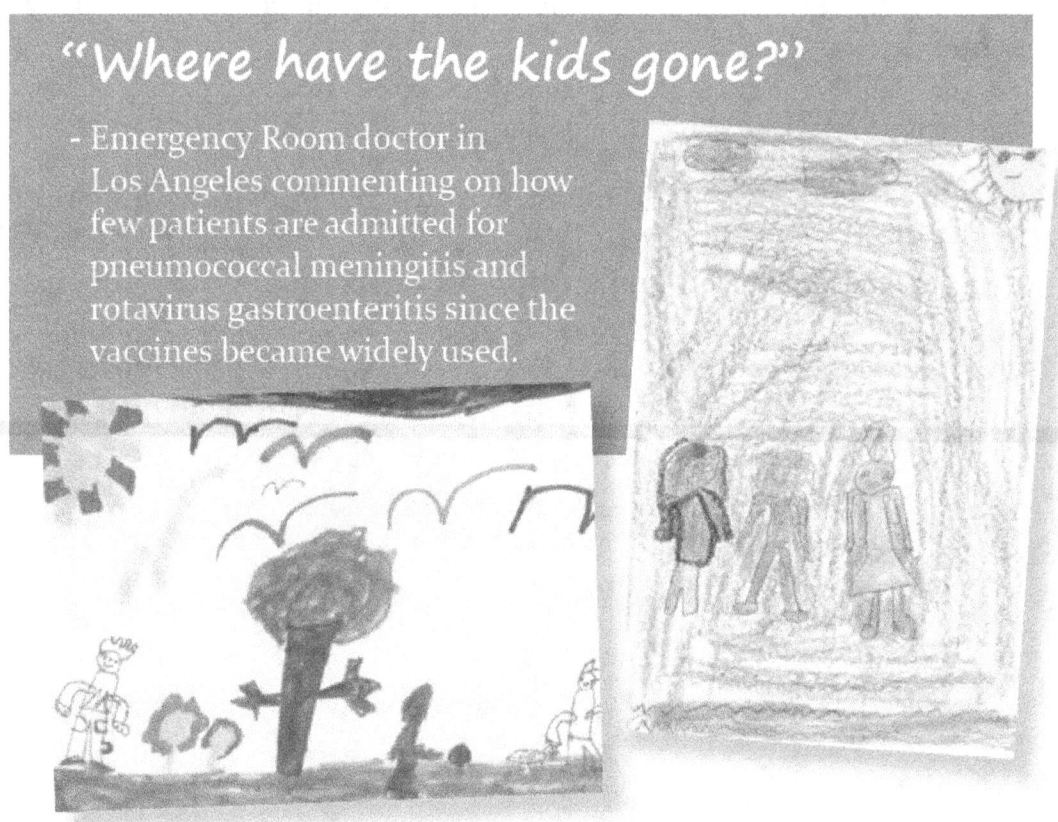

"Where have the kids gone?"

- Emergency Room doctor in Los Angeles commenting on how few patients are admitted for pneumococcal meningitis and rotavirus gastroenteritis since the vaccines became widely used.

Here are some examples of how much disease levels declined since vaccination began.

Disease	Annual Number of Reported Cases: Pre-Vaccine	Number of Reported Cases: 2007	Percent Decline
Diphtheria	175,885	0	100%
Tetanus	1,314	28	98%
Measles	503,282	43	99.9%
Mumps	152,209	800	99.5%
Rubella	47,745	12	99.9%
Congenital Rubella Syndrome	823	0	100%

The "pre-vaccine" figures are averages of reported cases, representing yearly incidence during the years just prior to the availability of a vaccine.

Vaccines

There are ten routine childhood vaccines that protect children from the 14 diseases described in this booklet:

DTaP: Protects against Diphtheria, Tetanus & Pertussis
MMR: Protects against Measles, Mumps & Rubella
HepA: Protects against Hepatitis A
HepB: Protects against Hepatitis B
Hib: Protects against *Haemophilus influenzae* type b
Flu: Protects against Influenza
PCV13: Protects against Pneumococcal disease
Polio: Protects against Polio
RV: Protects against Rotavirus
Varicella: Protects against Chickenpox

(Some bacteria or viruses – for example, pneumococcal, rotavirus, and influenza – have many strains, and existing vaccines protect only against selected strains . . . generally the most common or those most likely to cause illness in children.)

All of these vaccines are injections (shots), except for rotavirus, which is given orally, and one type of influenza vaccine, which is sprayed into the nose.

The Vaccine Schedule

All childhood vaccines are given as a series of 2 or more doses. The childhood vaccine schedule shows the recommended ages at which each vaccine dose should be given.

Here is the routine childhood schedule. For a more detailed and comprehensive version of this schedule, you can visit the CDC website at: **http://www.cdc.gov/vaccines/recs/schedules/default. htm#child**.

- For some of these vaccines, a booster dose at 4-6 years is also recommended.

- Influenza (flu) vaccine is recommended every winter for children 6 months of age and older.

at birth	HepB
2 months	HepB (1-2 mos) + DTaP + PCV13 + Hib + Polio + RV
4 months	DTaP + PCV13 + Hib + Polio + RV
6 months	HepB (6-18 mos) + DTaP + PCV13 + Hib + Polio (6-36 mos) + RV
12 Months	MMR (12-15 mos) + PCV13 (12-15 mos) + Hib (12-15 mos) + Varicella (12-15 mos) + HepA (12-23 mos)
15 months	DTaP (15-18 mos)

Flexibility in the Vaccine Schedule

Vaccine doses are recommended at specific ages. These recommendations are based on studies showing when children are at highest risk for the different diseases and at what ages vaccines work best. But the schedule is not "one size fits all," as it has been described by some people. It can be modified in several ways:

1. Notice that some of the doses on the above schedule may be given over a *range* of ages. For example, the 6-month dose of Polio vaccine can actually be given anywhere between 6 and 18 months without making it less effective.

2. A number of "combination" vaccines are also available. Combination vaccines contain several vaccines in a single injection. Combination vaccines include:
   DTaP-Polio-Hepatitis B (also called Pediarix®)
   DTaP-Hib (also called TriHIBit®)
   DTaP-Polio-Hib (also called Pentacel®)
   DTaP-Polio (also called Kinrix®)
   Hib-Hepatitis B (also called Comvax®)
   MMR-Varicella (also called MMRV or Proquad®)

3. Finally, for every vaccine there are "contraindications" and "precautions." These are conditions that make a child ineligible to get certain vaccines, or cause vaccine doses to be postponed. For example, a child who has a severe allergy to eggs should not get flu vaccine (which contains egg protein); or a child with a weakened immune system should not get live-virus vaccines. A child who is moderately or seriously ill should usually wait until he recovers before getting any vaccine.

You can talk with your doctor or nurse about using combination vaccines and taking advantage of the age ranges for certain vaccine doses to customize your baby's personal immunization schedule, reducing the number of shots she gets at a given visit. They will also help you determine if any contraindications or precautions apply to your baby.

Other Vaccines

In addition to these routine childhood vaccines, there are other vaccines that are recommended for older children or adolescents, or for young children under certain circumstances.

Rabies vaccine might be recommended for children bitten by animals, or for children living or traveling in a country where rabies is common.

Children traveling abroad may need other vaccines too, depending on the countries they are visiting. These vaccines could include Japanese encephalitis, Typhoid, Meningococcal, or Yellow fever.

Meningococcal vaccine is recommended for adolescents between 11 and 18 years of age and younger children with certain medical conditions to protect them from an infection that can cause bacterial meningitis. Tdap, a vaccine similar to DTaP, only formulated for adolescents and adults, is recommended at the 11-12 year doctor's visit. Human papillomavirus (HPV) vaccine is also recommended at 11-12 years of age.

Human papillomavirus is a major cause of cervical cancer.

Your health-care provider can advise you about the use of these vaccines.

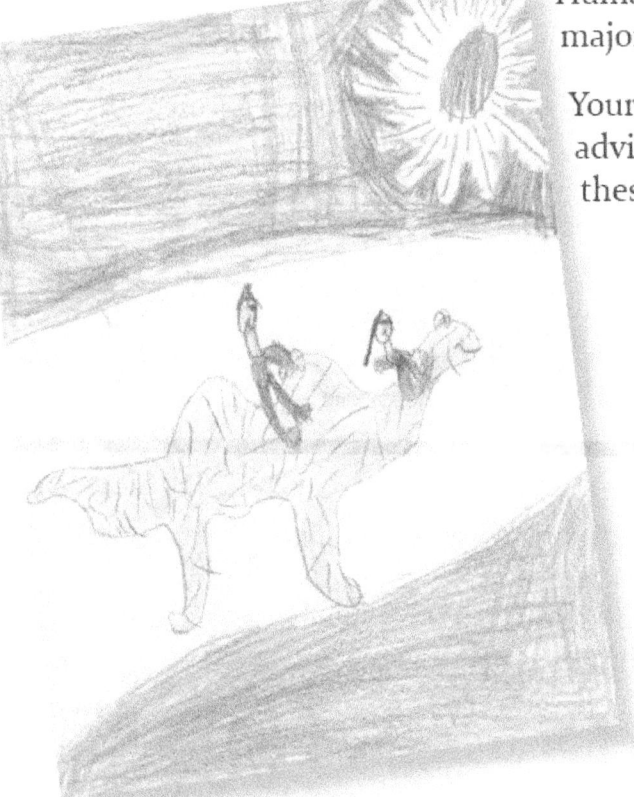

Vaccine Trivia:

The world's first vaccine, Dr. Edward Jenner's smallpox vaccine, was actually made from *cowpox* virus. Jenner called the process "vaccination" from *vacca*, a Latin word for cow.

Smallpox is the first, and so far the only, disease completely eradicated from the planet, thanks to vaccination. The last case of smallpox on Earth was in 1977.

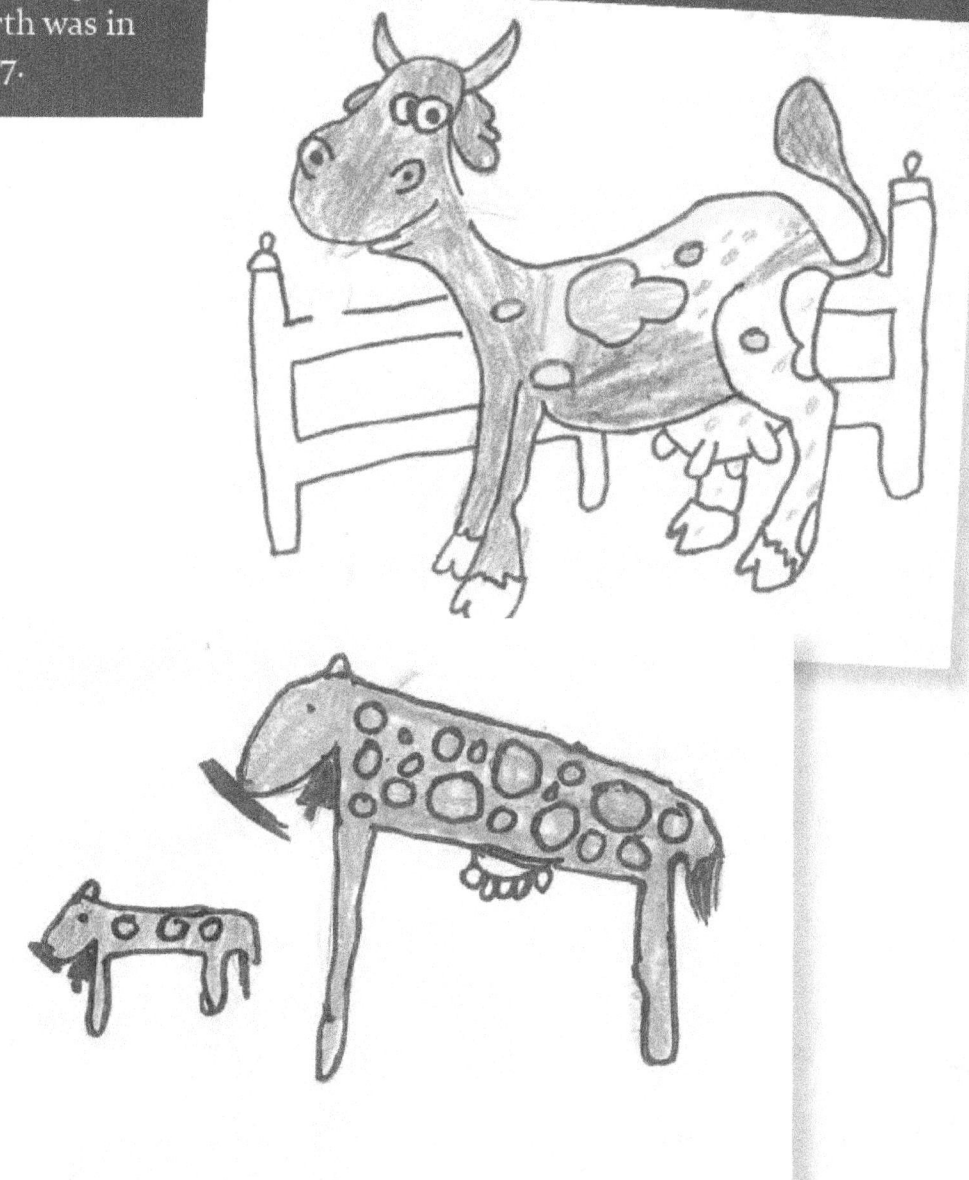

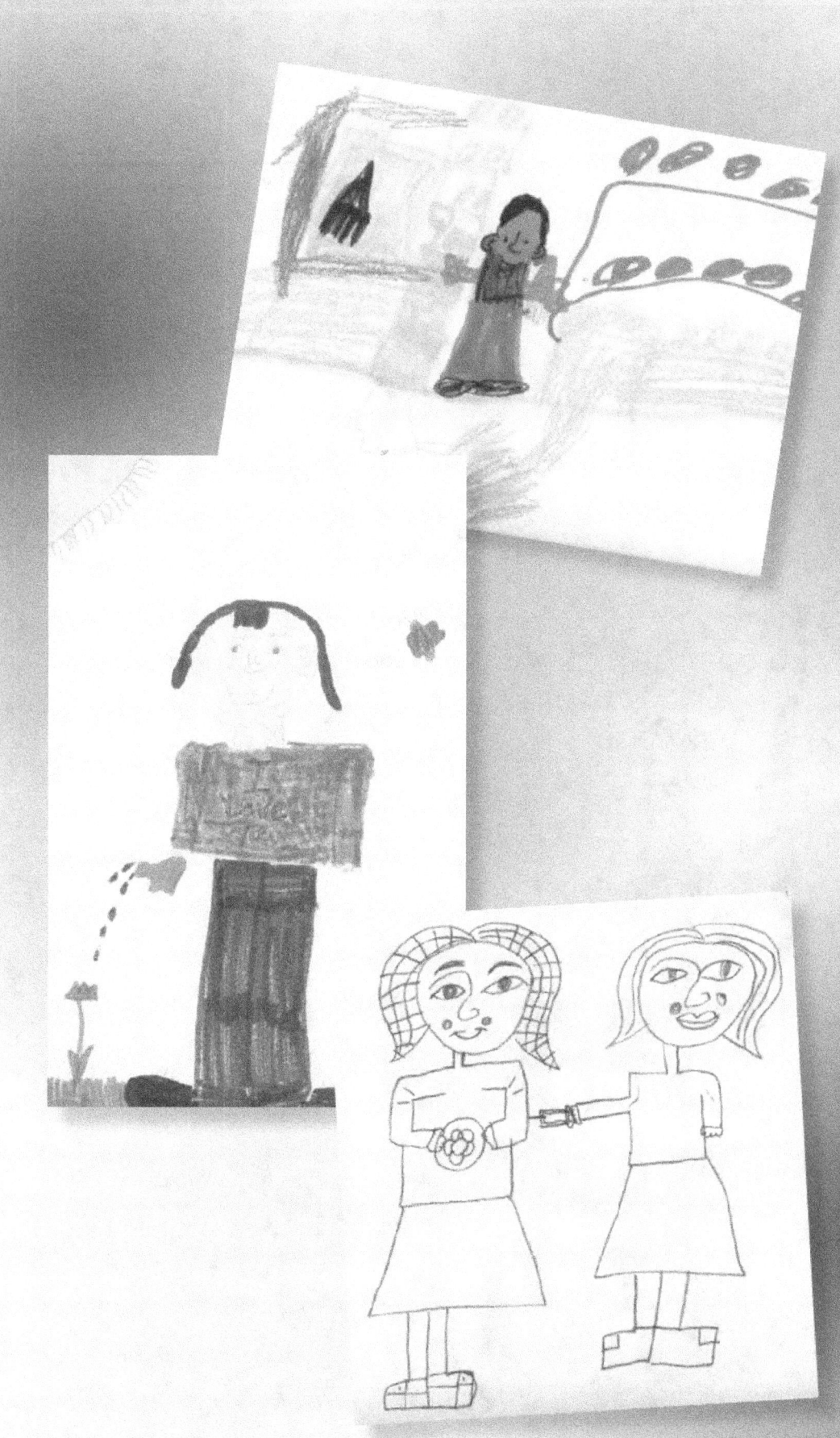

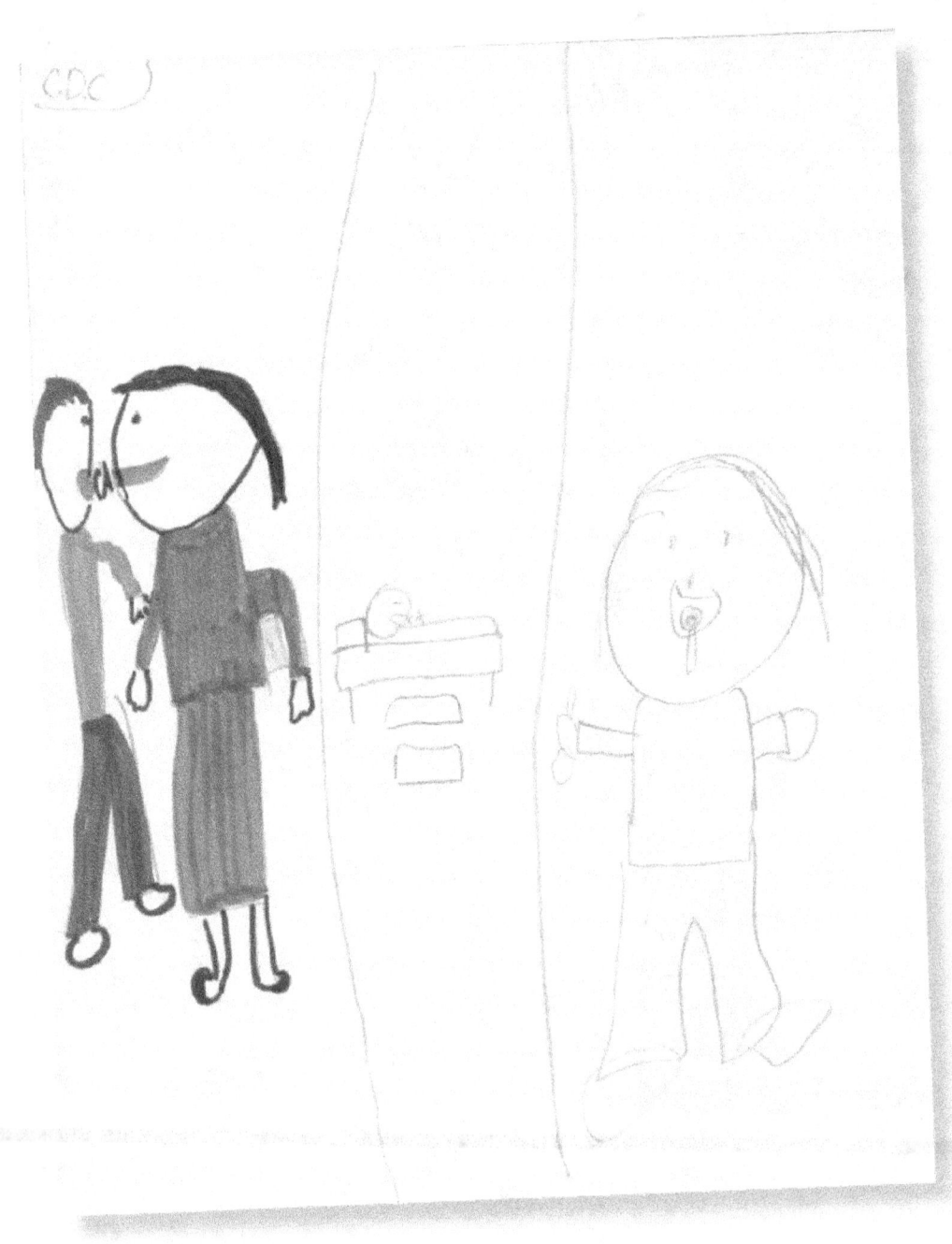

Parent's Guide to CHILDHOOD IMMUNIZATIONS

Part 2: The Immunization Office Visit

Before the Immunization Visit

If you have a vaccination record card for your baby, take it along so the provider can mark the shots given to her today. If she is getting her first vaccination(s), ask for a card. This record could come in handy later to show that your child has had the vaccinations necessary to get into school, or if you move or switch doctors.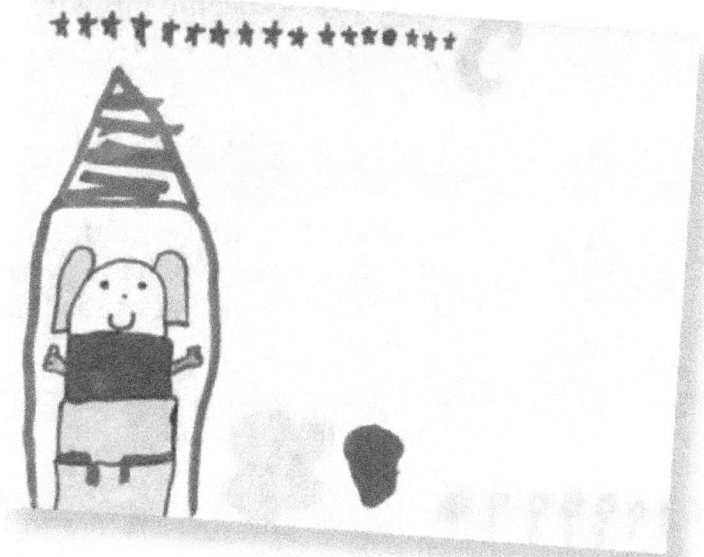

Your baby's vaccines may also be entered into an electronic registry, or "immunization information system."

The doctor or nurse will ask you some questions about your baby. Some of these questions will be to make sure there are no reasons your baby should not get certain vaccines. Be prepared to answer:

- Has your baby had a severe reaction to a previous dose of any vaccine?

  Babies often get a sore leg or a mild fever after vaccinations. But let your provider know if your baby has ever had a more serious side effect. There are a few uncommon reactions that could be a reason to not give another dose of a vaccine.

- Does your baby have any severe allergies?

  A baby who has a severe allergy to a substance that is in a vaccine shouldn't get that vaccine. (By a severe allergy we mean one that could be life-threatening. Less severe allergies aren't a problem.)

Naturally you can't be expected to know whether or not your baby is allergic to every substance in every vaccine. All you can do is report any allergies you do know about. Your doctor or nurse will be able to cross-check these against lists of vaccine ingredients.

Don't be too worried about allergies you don't know about. Severe allergic reactions to vaccines are rare (around 1 in a million), and your provider is prepared to deal with them if they do occur.

Among allergies that you might know about are eggs, gelatin and yeast, which are in certain vaccines, and latex, which might be part of the syringe or in the stopper of a vaccine vial.

-Does your child have an immune system problem?

A child with a suppressed immune system should not get certain (live) vaccines. A suppressed immune system can be caused by diseases such as AIDS, leukemia, or cancer, or by medical treatments such as steroids, chemotherapy, or radiation.

Your doctor, nurse, or other provider will be able to help you answer any questions.

During the Immunization Visit

Your provider should give you a Vaccine Information Statement (VIS) for each vaccine your child receives. The VIS contains useful information about the vaccine, including its risks and benefits. If you would like to review these statements before the office visit, you can find them online at **www.cdc.gov/vaccines/pubs/vis/default.htm**. There is a VIS for each vaccine, and many of them are also available in languages other than English.

Your provider will ask questions like those mentioned in the previous section, to determine if your baby has any contraindications or precautions to vaccination.

Always ask your provider if you have any questions or would like more information.

Your provider might ask you to hold your baby in a certain way to steady the arm or leg where the shot will be given. These techniques are designed to keep her still without actually holding her down or frightening her.

Many providers like to keep a child in the office for observation for about 15 or 20 minutes after getting vaccines, in the unlikely event of an allergic reaction or in case the child becomes dizzy or faints.

If your baby has a moderate or severe cold or other illness, you might be asked to postpone vaccinations until he gets better.

Be sure that any vaccinations that are given get recorded in your baby's shot record.

After the Immunization Visit

Sometimes a child will have a fever or a sore leg or arm (where the shot was given) after an immunization visit. You can give your child a non-aspirin pain reliever to reduce any pain or fever that might follow vaccinations. Giving the child plenty of fluids to drink can also help reduce a fever. A cool, wet washcloth over the sore area can help relieve pain.

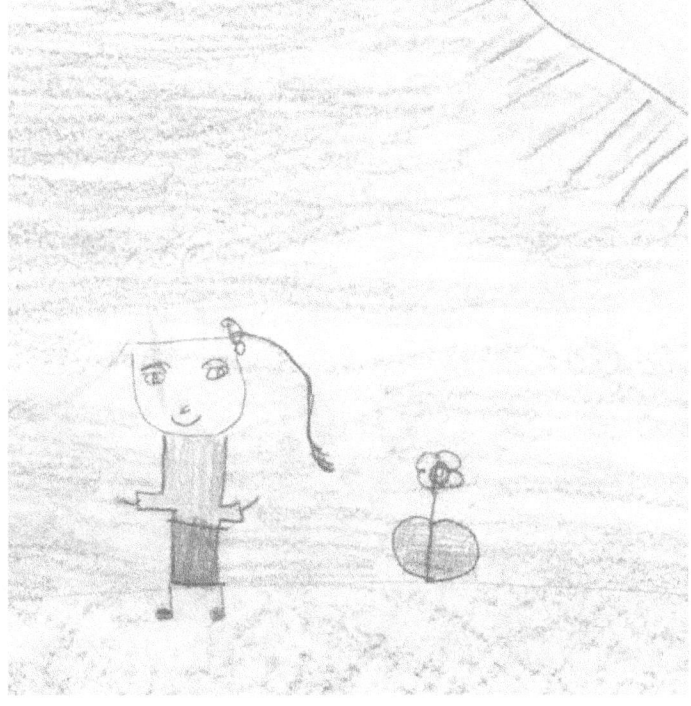

If your baby cries for 3 or more hours without quitting, if he seems limp or unresponsive, if he starts having seizures (convulsions), or if you are worried at all about how your baby looks or feels, call your provider right away. Serious reactions are uncommon, but your provider will know how to deal with them if they occur.

Once again, a severe allergic reaction to a vaccine is very unlikely, but if one were to occur, be ready to respond to it:

- If an allergic reaction occurs, it will usually happen within a few minutes to a few hours after the vaccination.

- Signs of a severe allergic reaction can include difficulty breathing, dizziness, swelling of the throat, hives, fast heartbeat, hoarseness or wheezing.

- If your baby shows these signs, **call a doctor and get him to a doctor right away.**

- Be ready to tell the doctor when the reaction occurred, what vaccinations were given, and when.

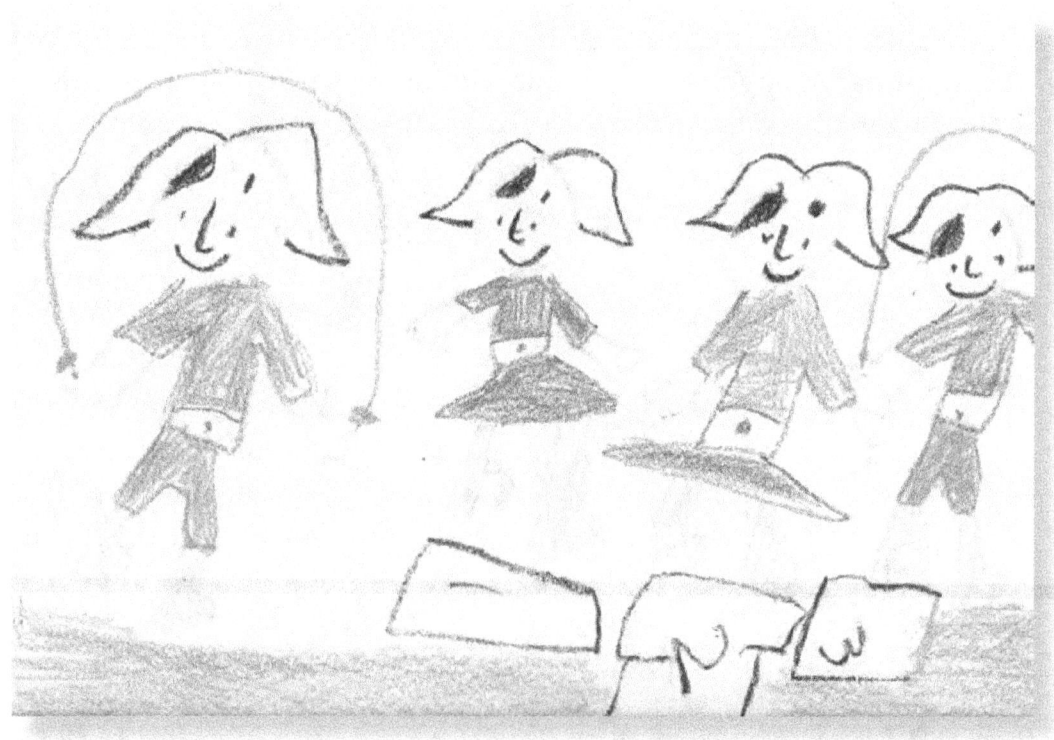

In the unlikely event that your child does have a serious reaction, first have it taken care of by your doctor or other provider. But afterward, there are two programs you should know about:

- **VAERS.** This stands for the **Vaccine Adverse Event Reporting System.** It is a system for reporting vaccine side effects. If your child has an unusual medical condition within a few days after getting a vaccine, even if you don't know whether it was caused by the vaccine, you should report it to VAERS. One of the jobs of VAERS is to collect these reports and use the data to help determine whether specific medical problems might be caused by vaccines.

  Your provider will usually file a VAERS report for you. However, you can also file it yourself. For more information, see the VAERS website at **www.vaers.hhs.gov**.

- **Vaccine Injury Compensation Program**. If you believe your child was seriously injured by a vaccine, there is a no-fault federal program that can help compensate you for his care.
  To learn more about the Vaccine Injury Compensation Program, see their website at **www.hrsa.gov/vaccinecompensation**.

Most parents will never need these programs, but they are there if you do.

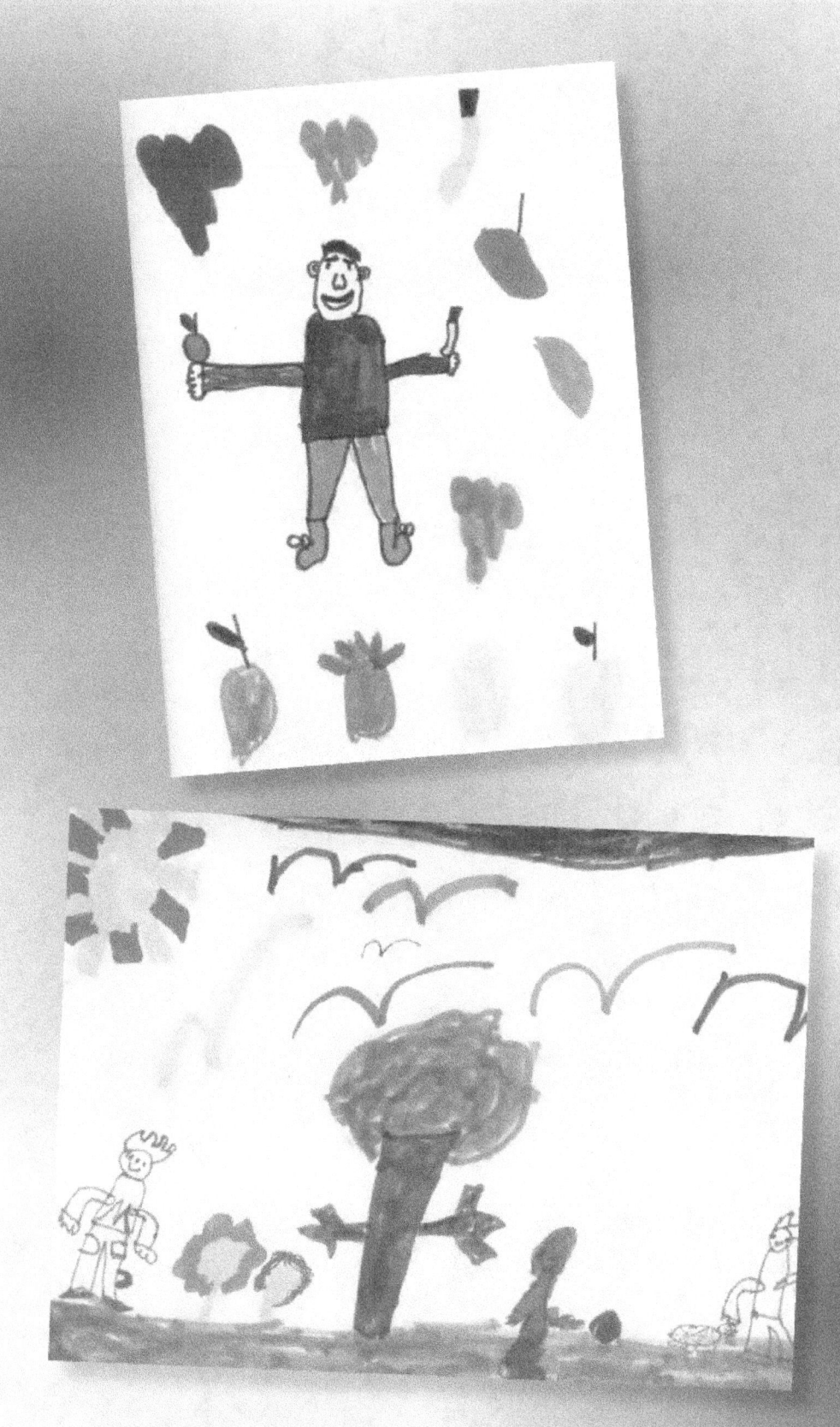

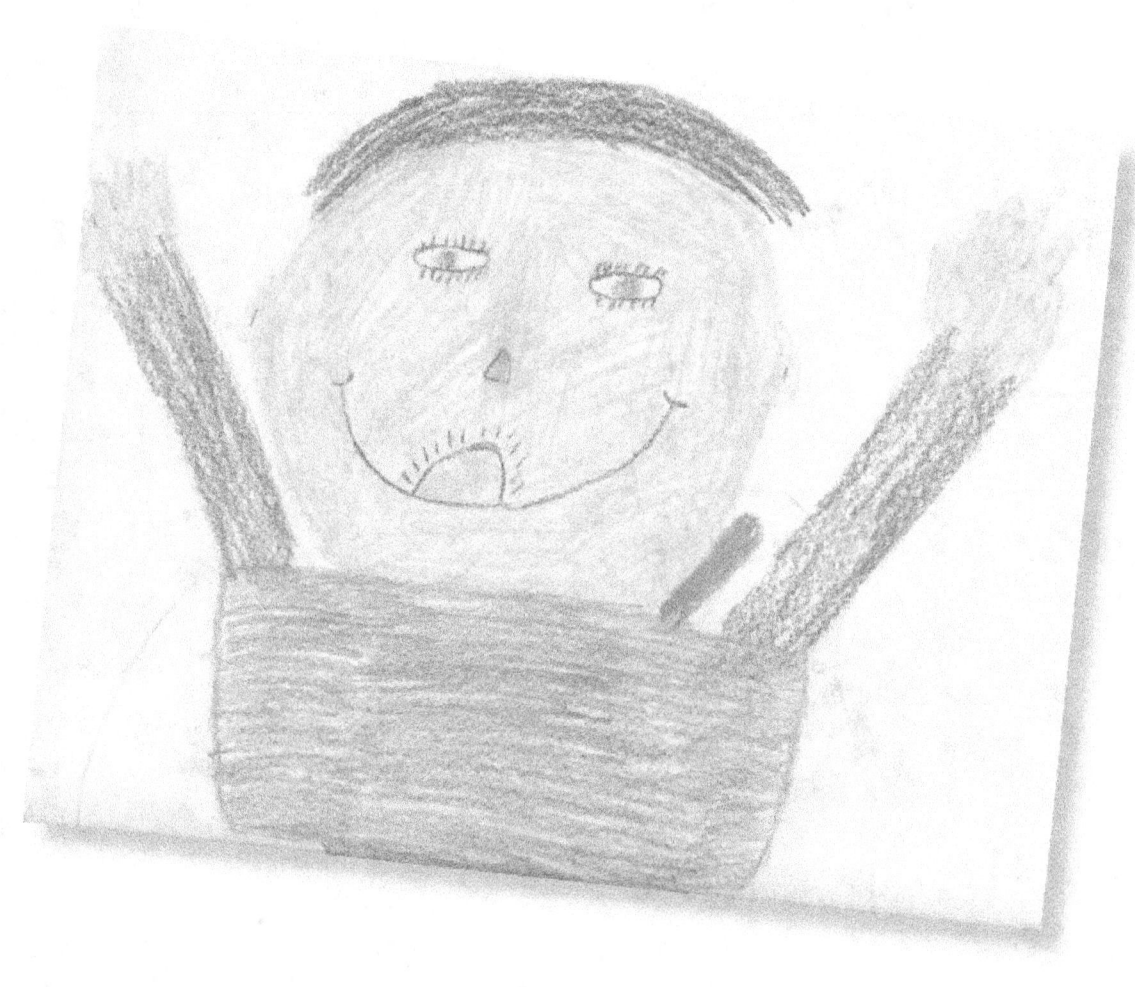

Parent's Guide to CHILDHOOD IMMUNIZATIONS

Part 3: More About Vaccines

How do vaccines work?

To understand how vaccines work, it helps to understand how immunity works.

Immunity

The human immune system is designed to protect us from anything that enters our body that doesn't belong there (not including food, of course). Immunologists call these things "non-self."

When a disease organism (that is, a germ – a virus or bacteria) enters the body, the immune system recognizes it as "non-self," and produces proteins called antibodies to get rid of it. These antibodies find and destroy the specific germ that is causing the infection. (For example, antibodies to polio attack polio virus and nothing else.)

But in addition, the immune system *remembers* this germ. Later on, if the person is exposed to the same germ again, antibodies are quickly deployed to eliminate it before it can make the person sick again. This is immunity.

Immunity is why a person who gets an infectious disease doesn't get the same disease again. (There are exceptions: many different viruses can cause the common cold, for example, and flu viruses change from year to year, so existing antibodies might not recognize them.)

This is a very efficient system. There is only one problem with it.

The first time a child is exposed to a disease, his immune system can't create antibodies quickly enough to keep him from getting sick. Eventually they will fight off the infection, and leave the child immune to future infections. But not before child gets sick with the disease.

In other words, the child has to get sick before becoming immune.

Vaccines

This problem is solved by vaccines. Vaccines contain the same germs that cause disease (for example, measles vaccine contains measles virus, and Hib vaccine contains Hib bacteria). But they have been either killed, or weakened to the point that they don't make you sick. Some vaccines contain only a *part* of the disease germ.

When a child is vaccinated, the vaccine stimulates his immune system to produce antibodies, exactly like it would if he were exposed to the disease. The child will develop immunity to that disease, and best of all he doesn't have to get sick first.

This is what makes vaccines such powerful medicine. Unlike most medicines, which treat or cure diseases, vaccines *prevent* them.

How *Well* Do Vaccines Work?

They work really well. No medicine is perfect, of course, but most childhood vaccines produce immunity about 90% to 100% of the time. (What about the small percent of children who don't develop immunity? We'll get to them later.)

But first, what about the argument made by some people that vaccines don't work that well . . . that diseases would be going away on their own because of better hygiene or sanitation, even if there were no vaccines?

That simply isn't true. Certainly better hygiene and sanitation can help prevent the spread of disease, but the germs that cause disease will still be around, and as long as they are they will continue to make people sick.

All vaccines are licensed by the Food and Drug Administration (FDA), and a vaccine must undergo extensive testing to show that it works and that it is safe before the FDA will approve it. Among these tests are *clinical trials*, which compare groups of people who get a vaccine with groups of people who don't. Unless the vaccinated groups are much less likely to get the disease, the vaccine won't be licensed.

If you look at the history of any vaccine-preventable disease, you will virtually always see that the number of cases of disease starts to drop when a vaccine is licensed. Here's a chart showing this pattern for measles:

Measles - United States, 1950-2007

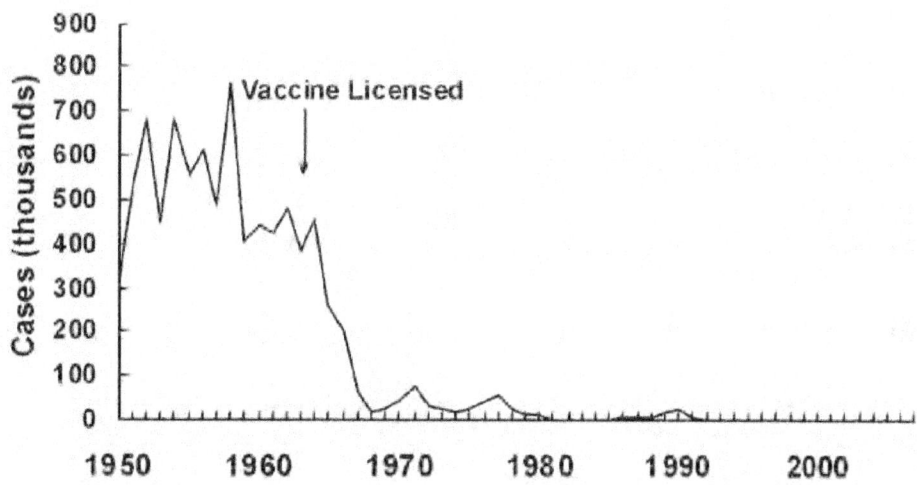

Measles vaccine was licensed in 1962, and as you can see, that's when the number of cases started to decline. (Measles didn't completely disappear after 1993; there have just been too few cases to show up on this graph.)

If the drop in disease were due to hygiene and sanitation, you would expect all diseases to start going away at about the same time. But if you were to look at the graph for polio, for example, you would see the number of cases start to drop around 1955 – the year the first polio vaccine was licensed. If you look at the graph for Hib, the number drops around 1990, for pneumococcal disease around 2000 — corresponding to the introduction of vaccines for those diseases.

How Safe Are Vaccines?

This is a question that will naturally concern any new parent. No matter how good vaccines are at preventing disease, no matter how much they have reduced disease over the years, no matter how many lives they have saved, what if they can actually harm my baby?

Vaccine safety is a complex issue. We will address some specific safety issues in the Frequently Asked Questions section of this booklet (page 43). In the meantime, here are some general facts:

Can vaccines harm my child? Any medicine can cause a reaction, even aspirin. Vaccines are no exception.

Will vaccines harm my child? Probably not. Most children won't have any reaction at all to a given vaccine. For those who do, most reactions are very minor . . . a sore leg, a slight rash, or a mild fever that goes away within a day or two.

Some children have moderate reactions like a high fever, chills, or muscle aches.

One of the scariest of these reactions is called a *febrile seizure*. This is a seizure, or convulsion, caused by a high fever. During a febrile seizure a child might shake uncontrollably, become unresponsive, or even lose consciousness. About one child in 25 will have at least one febrile seizure during his childhood, usually between the ages of 6 months and 3 years. They often accompany ear infections or respiratory infections. When a febrile seizure is associated with a vaccine, it is because the vaccine causes a fever, which in turn triggers the seizure. While febrile seizures look serious, fortunately they almost never are. You can learn more about febrile seizures at **www.ninds.nih.gov/disorders/febrile_seizures/detail_febrile_seizures.htm**.

Rarely, a child may have a truly severe reaction, like encephalopathy (brain infection), or a severe allergic reaction. These are the scary possibilities that make some parents think that it might actually be better not to vaccinate their children. Would it?

First, severe reactions are extremely rare.

Second, it is sometimes hard to tell whether a reaction was actually caused by a vaccine. Any serious reaction that could be caused by a vaccine could also be caused by something else. There are no serious health problems caused only by vaccines. For something that affects only one child in a hundred thousand or a million, it can be very hard to isolate the cause.

Example: Some people used to believe DTP* vaccine caused Sudden Infant Death Syndrome (SIDS), citing as evidence lists of cases of SIDS that occurred one or two days after the DTP shot. But SIDS always occurs during the same age range when millions of babies get their routine shots, so it would be remarkable if SIDS *didn't* occasionally strike right after the shot. When scientists conducted controlled studies to test this theory they found that babies recently vaccinated with DTP were no more likely to get SIDS than those who weren't vaccinated. Subsequently, precautions such as putting babies to sleep on their backs have been found to dramatically reduce the risk of SIDS. (For more information about vaccines and SIDS, see **www.cdc.gov/vaccinesafety/Concerns/sids.html**.)

*DTP is an older version of DTaP.

Third, risk doesn't exist in a vacuum. You can't evaluate the risks of vaccination without also considering its benefits.

The risk from a vaccine is the chance it will cause a child serious harm. This risk is extremely small. Even a life-threatening allergic reaction can be brought under control by the trained staff in a doctor's office. For a summary of risks associated with a particular vaccine, you can read the Vaccine Information Statement for that vaccine – these can be found online at **www.cdc.gov/vaccines/pubs/vis/default.htm**.

The most obvious benefit of vaccination is, of course, protection from disease. But there is more to it than that. There are really three types of benefit to vaccination — **personal** benefits, **community** benefits, and **future** benefits. It is worth looking at each of these separately:

a) Personal benefits.

Vaccinating your child will protect him from a dozen or so potentially serious diseases.

But how likely is it that your child will actually get one of these diseases? Remember that vaccine-preventable diseases have been declining (thanks to vaccines), and that many of them are now at all-time lows. If the risk of disease is very low, isn't the benefit of vaccination also very low?

Good question. Statistically, the chance of *your* child getting a vaccine-preventable disease may be relatively low. You are making a wager.
If you choose vaccination you are betting that your child could be exposed to disease, so you accept the tiny risk of a serious vaccine reaction to protect him if that happens.

If you choose *not* to vaccinate, you are betting that your child probably *won't* be exposed to disease, or if he is, his illness won't be serious, and you are willing to accept the small risk of serious illness to avoid the small possibility of a vaccine reaction.

In our opinion, vaccinating is by far the safer bet. Even though diseases have declined, they haven't disappeared. A recent study showed that children who had not gotten DTaP vaccine were *23 times* more likely to get whooping cough than children who had. Thirty-one children died from whooping cough in 2005. That might not be many, but the number wouldn't matter if your child were one of them.

b) Community benefits.

Back on page 32 we said that a small percentage of children fail to develop immunity from vaccines. There are also children who cannot get certain vaccines for medical or other reasons, and those who are too young to be vaccinated.   These children have no protection if they are exposed to someone who is infected with a communicable disease.

When most children in a community are immune, even if one child gets sick, the disease will probably not spread. That's because it will have nowhere to go – if the sick child comes in contact only with children who are immune, the disease will die out. This is called *herd immunity*.

But when fewer children in a community are immune, it is easier for a disease to spread from person to person and cause an outbreak. As this booklet was being written, Wales was experiencing a "massive" measles outbreak because of parents' failure to vaccinate their children. And outbreaks of measles, mumps, and whooping cough are occurring around the United States – often among groups of children whose parents have refused to get them vaccinated. Recently in California, a boy who contracted measles during a European vacation came back and infected 11 of his unvaccinated classmates.

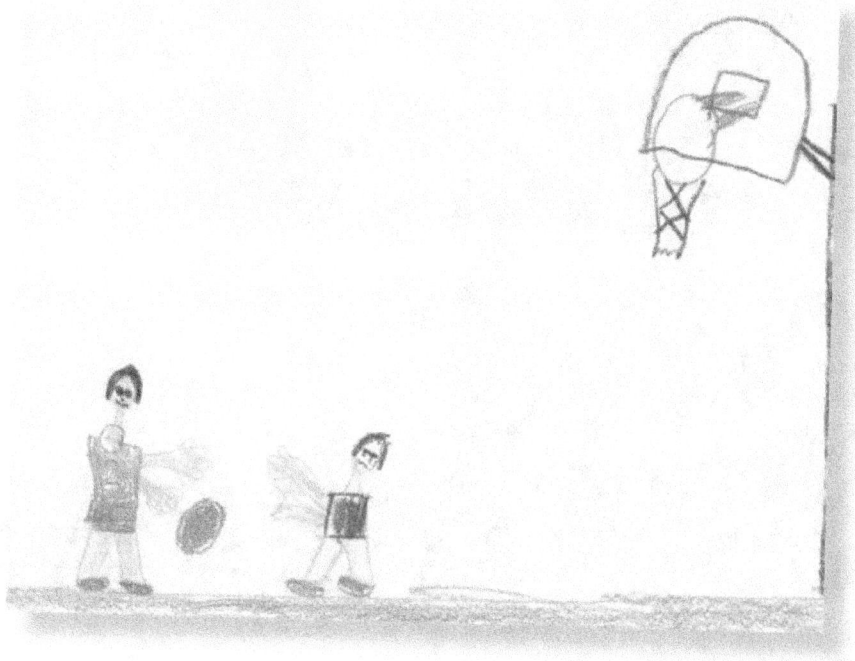

Meet Riley

In most ways Riley is a typical eight-year-old girl. She takes piano and gymnastics lessons, plays soccer, likes to swim, and gets into fights with her brothers.

But Riley has something most eight-year olds don't – another child's heart. She was born with a serious heart defect and had to get a transplant within days of her birth.

To Riley's immune system, her new heart doesn't belong, because it is "non-self," like a disease germ (see page 31). Her immune system would reject it if she didn't take special drugs. These drugs suppress her immune system, and because of this she can't get live-virus vaccines like measles, mumps, rubella, or chickenpox.

Consequently, Riley is not immune to these diseases. She has to depend on the immunity of people around her for protection. If one of her schoolmates or playmates were to come down with a case of measles or chicken-pox, Riley could easily catch it from them. And because her immune system can't fight off the infection, it could become very serious if not treated promptly.

Riley enjoys a normal life today, partly thanks to her friends who are protecting her from infections by getting all their shots.

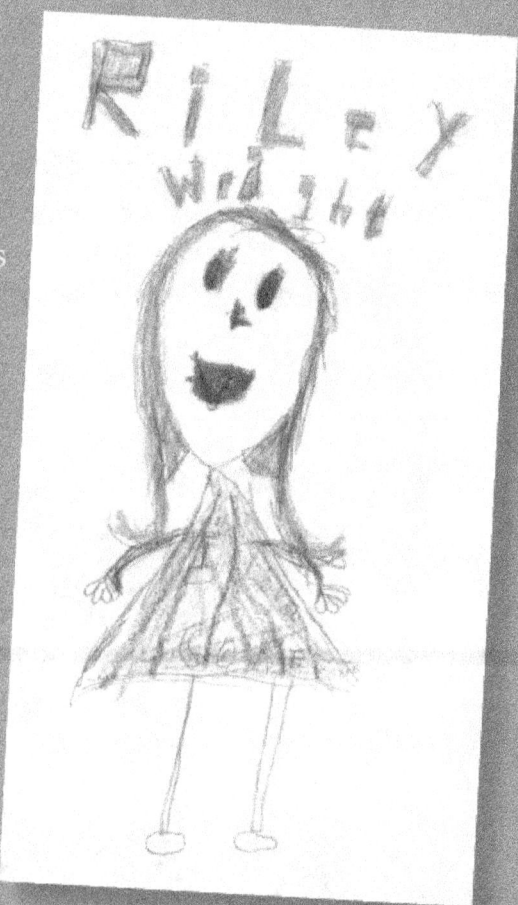

Riley's self-portrait

In other words, you are not just protecting your own child by getting her vaccinated, you are protecting other children – adults too.

c) Future benefits.

Rates of vaccine-preventable diseases are very low in the United States. So the risk of an individual child getting, say, a case of measles is very low too. What would happen, then, if we all just stopped vaccinating? We know what would happen because we have seen it in other countries. Diseases that have been declining for years would come back.

> Example: In the mid-1970s, most Japanese children (about 80%) got pertussis vaccine. In 1974 there were only 393 cases of whooping cough in the entire country, and no one died from it.
> But then, because of a scare about the vaccine's safety, the immunization rate dropped to only about 10% over the next few years. By 1979 the country was in the grip of a whooping cough epidemic that infected more than 13,000 people and left 41 dead that year. When routine vaccination was resumed, the disease numbers dropped again.

The point is, we can't stop vaccinating, because even though disease rates are low, they are not zero. Even a few cases in a vulnerable population could touch off a major outbreak. This is why we still vaccinate against polio, even though we haven't seen it in this country for more than 10 years. One infected traveler from a country where polio *hasn't* been eliminated could set us back 50 years if our own population wasn't protected.

To summarize: When you vaccinate your child, you are not just protecting her. You are also protecting her friends and schoolmates and their families; and you are also protecting her children, her grandchildren, and all future generations.

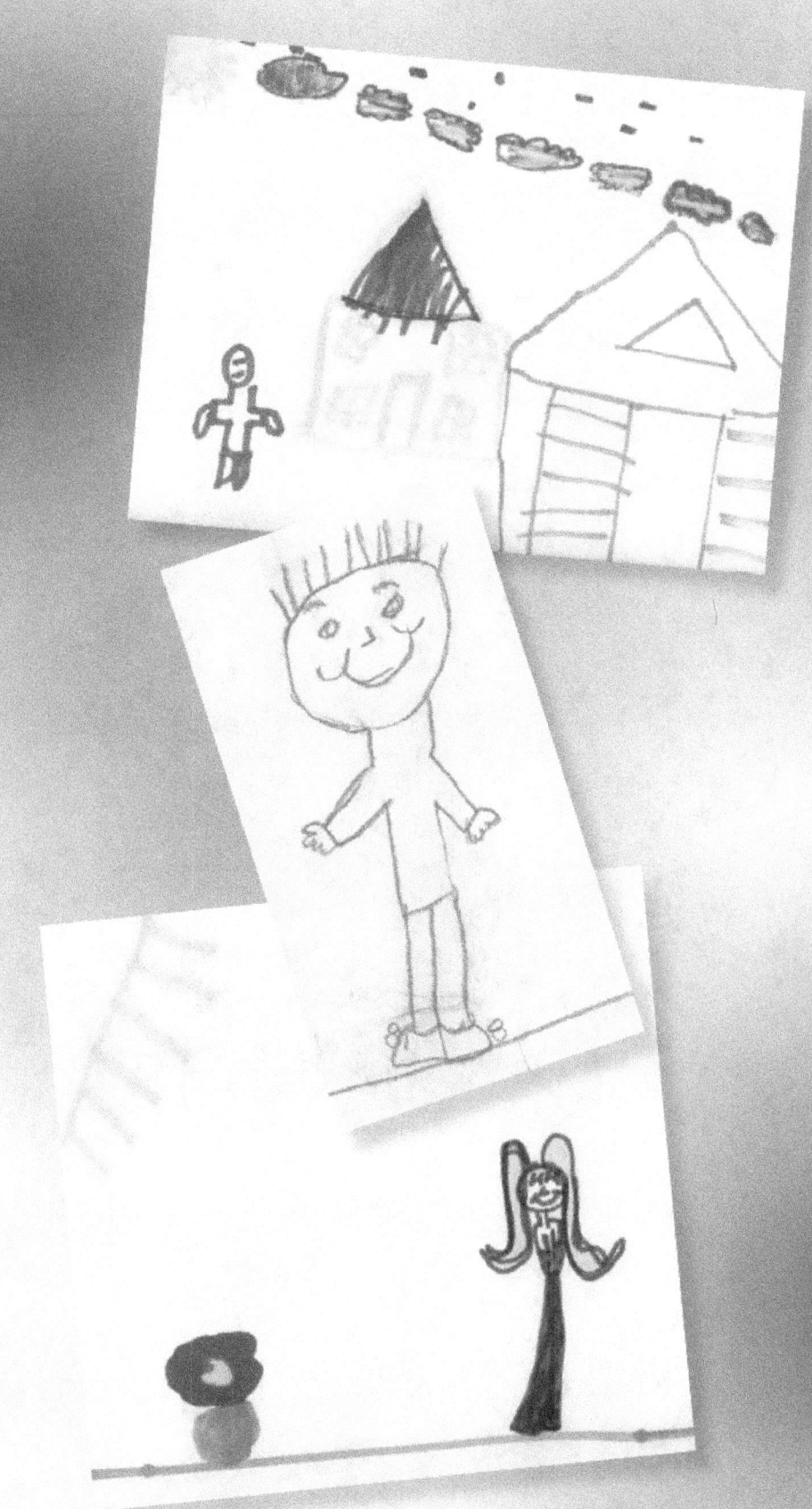

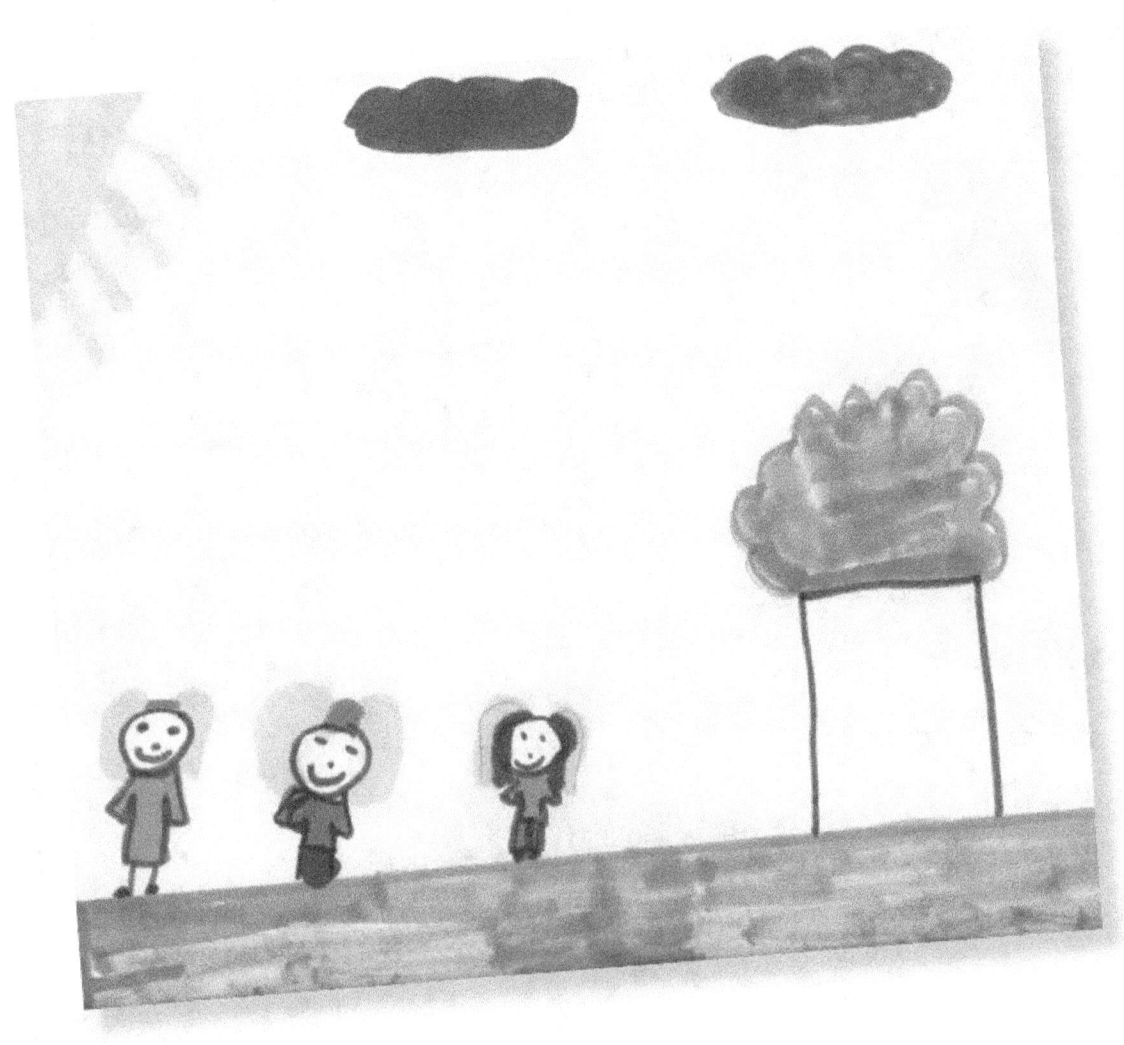

Parent's Guide to CHILDHOOD IMMUNIZATIONS

Part 4: Frequently Asked Questions

How can we be sure vaccines don't cause long-term problems?

Tracking vaccinated children for many years looking for long-term health conditions would be impractical; and withholding new vaccines from children who would benefit from them while long-term studies were being done would be unethical. A more practical approach is to look at the conditions themselves, and at the factors that cause them. Scientists are already working constantly to identify risk factors that can lead to conditions like cancer, stroke, heart disease, and autoimmune diseases like lupus or rheumatoid arthritis. Thousands of studies have already been done looking at hundreds of potential risk factors. If immunizations were identified as a risk factor in any of these studies, we would immediately know about it. So far, they have not.

We know vaccines' safety record from clinical trials before they were licensed, and from millions of doses administered after they were licensed. And we know there is no plausible biologic reason to believe vaccines would cause any serious long-term effects. Based on more than 50 years of experience with vaccines, we can say that the likelihood that a vaccine will cause unanticipated long-term problems is extremely low.

In addition, every vaccine is continually monitored for safety. If an unexpected problem were detected at any time, it would be dealt with appropriately.

> Example: The first vaccine for rotavirus was licensed in 1998. Within a year, monitoring systems (like VAERS) revealed that a type of intestinal blockage called intussusception was occurring in children who got the vaccine slightly more often than it would have been expected to occur by chance. This was too uncommon to have been detected during clinical trials, and was only apparent after millions of children had been vaccinated. Once the problem was detected, the vaccine was immediately taken off the market.
>
> (Two new rotavirus vaccines are now available, neither of which has been associated with intussusception, even after intensive scrutiny.)

If all my child's friends are vaccinated, won't he be protected by herd immunity? Why should I put <u>my</u> child at risk for vaccine reactions if all the other children around him are already immune?

This is like riding in a car pool where everyone contributes each month to pay for gas, repairs to the car, etc.; and one morning a new guy shows up and says, "I think I'll ride along with you. But I'm not going to pay, since you're going downtown anyway and you have an empty seat." If enough people choose to take a free ride on other children's immunity, herd immunity will soon disappear.

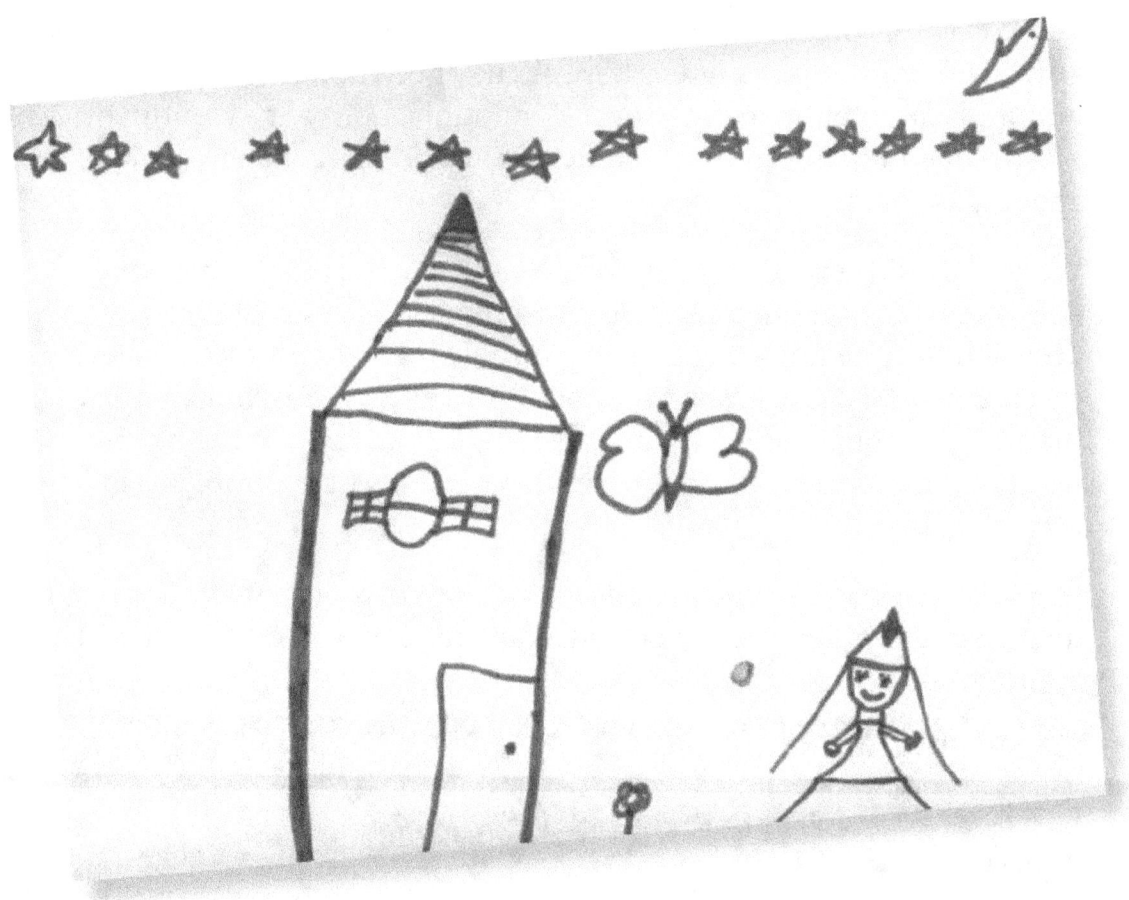

Why do children need so many doses of certain vaccines?

Most vaccines require at least 2 doses. With inactivated (killed) vaccines, each dose of vaccine contains a fixed amount of disease antigen (virus or bacteria). Immunity is built in phases with each dose boosting immunity to a protective level. Live vaccines are " different, in that the antigen in the vaccine reproduces and spreads throughout the body. One dose produces satisfactory immunity in most children. But a second dose is given to assure immunity, because not all children respond to the first one.

What is in vaccines?

Vaccines contain several basic types of substances:

1. All vaccines contain disease antigen – in other words a killed or weakened form of the disease germ that the vaccine protects against. Disease antigen is the core of any vaccine; it is the part that produces immunity.

2. Some vaccines contain **adjuvants**. These are substances that help vaccines produce a stronger immune response.

3. Some vaccines come in vials containing multiple doses. Some of these contain a **preservative**, to prevent contamination once the vial has been opened.

4. A **diluent** is a liquid – usually saline or sterile water – used to reconstitute a powdered vaccine.

5. Vaccine antigens are grown on "growth media" that can contain a variety of substances, such as yeast. Other substances, such as formaldehyde, can be used during the production of vaccines. All these substances are removed from the final product, but tiny traces of them, too small to have a clinical effect, can remain.

Aren't some of these substances toxic?

Some vaccine ingredients could be toxic . . . *at much higher doses.* This concerns some parents, but the fact is that any substance – even water – can be toxic given a large enough dose. But at a very low dose, even a highly toxic substance can be safe.

We might not be aware of it, but we are exposed to small amounts of these same "toxic" substances every day. For example:

Mercury: Babies are exposed to mercury in milk, including breast milk. Seafood also contains mercury.

Formaldehyde: Formaldehyde is in automobile exhaust; in household products and furnishings such as carpets, upholstery, cosmetics, paint, and felt-tip markers; and in health products such as antihistamines, cough drops, and mouthwash.

Aluminum: The average person takes in an estimated 30 to 50 mg of aluminum every day, mainly from foods, drinking water, and medicines. Not all vaccines contain aluminum, but those that do typically contain about .125 mg to .625 mg per dose, or roughly 1% of that daily average.

One final word – don't believe everything you read about harmful ingredients in vaccines. To debunk just one popular myth, NO vaccine contains, or has ever contained, even a molecule of antifreeze. But if you search the web you can easily find a dozen websites that persist in claiming that they do.

Can a child get a disease even after being vaccinated?

It isn't very common, but it can happen.

About 1% to 5% of the time, depending on the vaccine, a child who is vaccinated fails to develop immunity. If these children are exposed to that disease they could get sick. Sometimes giving an additional vaccine dose will stimulate an immune response in a child who didn't respond to one dose. For example, a single dose of measles vaccine protects about 95% of children, but after two doses almost 100% are immune.

Sometimes a child is exposed to a disease just prior to being vaccinated, and gets sick before the vaccine has time to work.

Sometimes a child gets sick with something that is similar to a disease they have been vaccinated against. This often happens with flu. Many viruses cause symptoms that look like flu, and people even call some of them flu, even though they are really not. Flu vaccine doesn't protect from these viruses.

Can a child actually get the disease from a vaccine?

Almost never. With inactivated (killed) vaccines, it isn't possible. A dead virus or bacteria, or part of a virus or bacteria, can't cause disease.

With live vaccines, some children get what appears to be a mild case of disease (for example what looks like a measles or chickenpox rash but with only a few spots). This isn't harmful, and can actually show that the vaccine is working.

A vaccine causing full-blown disease would be extremely unlikely. One exception was the live oral polio vaccine, which could very rarely mutate and actually cause a case of polio. This was a rare but tragic side effect of this otherwise effective vaccine. Oral polio vaccine is no longer used in the U.S.

Why does the government require children to be vaccinated to attend school?

School immunization laws are not imposed by the federal government, but by the individual states. But that doesn't answer the question, which is often asked by people who see this as a violation of their individual rights.

The mission of a public health system, as its name implies, is to protect the health of the public – that is, everybody. Remember that vaccines protect not only the person being vaccinated but also people around them. Immunization laws exist not only to protect individual children, but to protect *all* children.

If vaccines were not mandatory, fewer people would get their children vaccinated – they would forget; they would put it off; they would feel they couldn't afford it; they wouldn't have time. This would lead to levels of immunity dropping below what are needed for herd immunity (see page 37), which would lead in turn to outbreaks of disease. So mandatory vaccination, while it might not be a perfect solution, is at least a practical solution to a difficult problem.

In a sense, school immunization laws are like traffic laws. We're not allowed to drive as fast as we want on crowded streets or to disobey traffic signals. This could be seen as an imposition on individual rights too. However, these laws are not so much to prevent drivers from harming themselves, which you could argue is their right, but to prevent them from harming others, which is not.

Can children be exempted from school immunization laws?

Under certain circumstances, yes. All states allow medical exemptions, so children who cannot safely receive certain vaccines (like Riley . . . see page 38) are not required to get them. Most states also allow religious exemptions for children whose religion prohibits vaccination. Finally, some states allow philosophic exemptions for people who oppose vaccination on non-religious grounds. To protect themselves and others, unvaccinated students may be prohibited from attending classes if there is an outbreak of a vaccine-preventable disease at their school or in their community.

Vaccines are expensive. Is there a way to reduce the cost?

You can go to a public clinic or health department rather than to a private physician. Vaccinations are generally cheaper there, and may be free except for an administration charge.

There is also a national program called Vaccines for Children (or VFC) that allows qualified families to get free vaccinations for their children at participating doctors' offices. You can learn more about the VFC program at **www.cdc.gov/vaccines/programs/vfc/default.htm**.

Can't so many vaccines overwhelm a child's immune system?

There may not be consensus over exactly how many germs a baby's immune system can handle at a time, but it is considerably more than they will ever get from vaccines. After all, this is the immune system's job. From the day a baby is born, her immune system is busy dealing with the thousands of germs she is exposed to as part of daily life. As one doctor put it, "Worrying about too many vaccines is like worrying about a thimble of water getting you wet when you are swimming in an ocean."

There are mothers who say that their babies developed autism after receiving their shots. If the shots didn't cause the autism, how do you explain this?

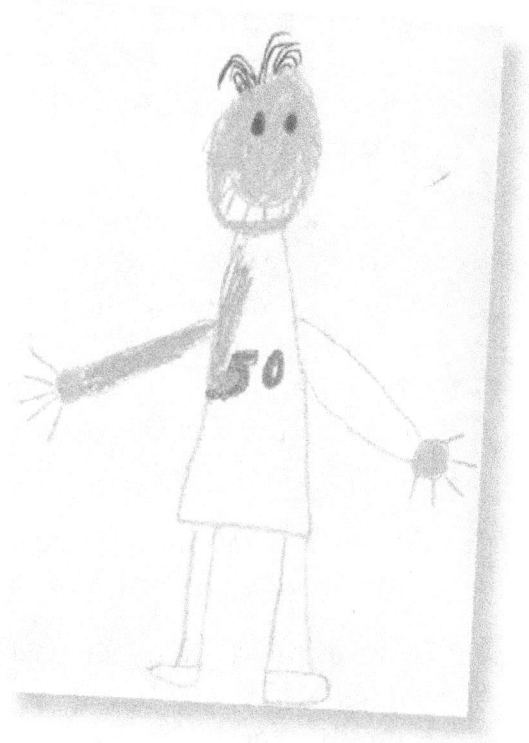

A parent's desire to know exactly why something as serious as autism has struck her child is very strong. The fact is, science has not yet determined exactly what causes autism. But parents can be reluctant to accept a "we don't know" answer when vaccines offer an easy and fairly plausible alternative.

Nevertheless, there *are* explanations.

First, remember the discussion about DTP vaccine and SIDS on page 35? The same explanation applies to vaccines and autism. Autism is usually diagnosed during the same age range when children are getting their routine shots. Naturally, if enough children develop autism during these ages, sometimes it will be noticed within a day or two after a vaccination visit. Even if it happens several hundred times, this is a tiny number compared with the millions of children who get vaccines every year and don't develop autism afterward.

Also, it is a very common logical error to assume that because one event directly follows another, it must have been caused by it. We laugh at the old folk belief that the rooster's crowing makes the sun come up, but the reasoning is exactly the same. The difference is that the idea of a rooster causing the sun to rise is ridiculous, while the idea that vaccines can cause autism sort of makes sense. But that doesn't make the argument any more valid. For the theory that vaccines cause autism to make logical sense, someone would have to show that children who get vaccinated are more likely to develop autism than children who don't. And no one has done that.

Why do you use vague language like, "Available data suggest that there is no association between vaccines and autism . . . ?" Why can't you just say, "Vaccines don't cause autism!" If your statements didn't sound so wishy-washy, they would be more believable.

It would be nice to simply say that vaccines don't cause autism, but it wouldn't be good science. A basic principle of science is that *you can't prove that something is not true*. We all believe that if you let go of an apple it will drop to the ground. But that belief is based on the observation that it has always happened that way in the past. It doesn't *prove* that the next time you try it, the apple might not fly up into the air instead.

So to say that vaccines don't cause autism would be scientifically dishonest, regardless of how sure we are that they don't.

What we *can* say is that at least a dozen rigorous scientific studies – designed to detect a connection between vaccines and autism – have been published in reputable, peer-reviewed journals; and these studies have overwhelmingly *failed to show any connection between vaccines and autism*. The Institute of Medicine, an independent, objective "advisor to the nation" on health, reviewed these studies, and concluded that there is no plausible evidence that vaccines cause autism. But they went farther than that. They advised that money that could be used to fund more studies on vaccines and autism would be better spent on areas of autism research more likely to be productive.

This isn't exactly saying, "Vaccines don't cause autism," but it is about as close as any group of scientists is likely to come to it.

How do you explain the increase in the number of children with autism, and the fact that the increase corresponded with an increase in the number of vaccinations children get?

The rise in the number of autism cases can be explained, at least in large part, by the fact that autism is being recognized and diagnosed much more often than it used to be, and that many conditions that used to go by other names are now being called autism, or autism spectrum disorder. The number of autism cases may actually be rising, but much of the apparent increase can be accounted for by the fact that we simply recognize it more often.

As for the correspondence between the rise in autism and the increase in the number of vaccinations, remember . . . just because one event preceded another, it doesn't mean it caused it. No one has proven that vaccines cause autism, and in fact virtually all reliable evidence says that they don't.

While there is evidence that genetics plays an important role in the development of autism, that doesn't necessarily rule out the possibility that environmental factors could play a role too. But even if this is true, why would it have to be vaccines? Many things in our society were changing at the same time more vaccines were being developed, from the amount of fast foods and processed foods we eat, to the amount of television we watch, to the amounts of industrial pollution we're exposed to, to other drugs and medicines we take, to chemicals in the clothes we wear and the homes we live in, to the amount of time we spend talking on cell phones – and that's just a few. You could list just as many more.

The theory that vaccines cause autism has been extensively tested, and has come up short. Maybe the Institute of Medicine is right, and it's time to devote more time and money looking into other, more promising, theories into the causes of autism.

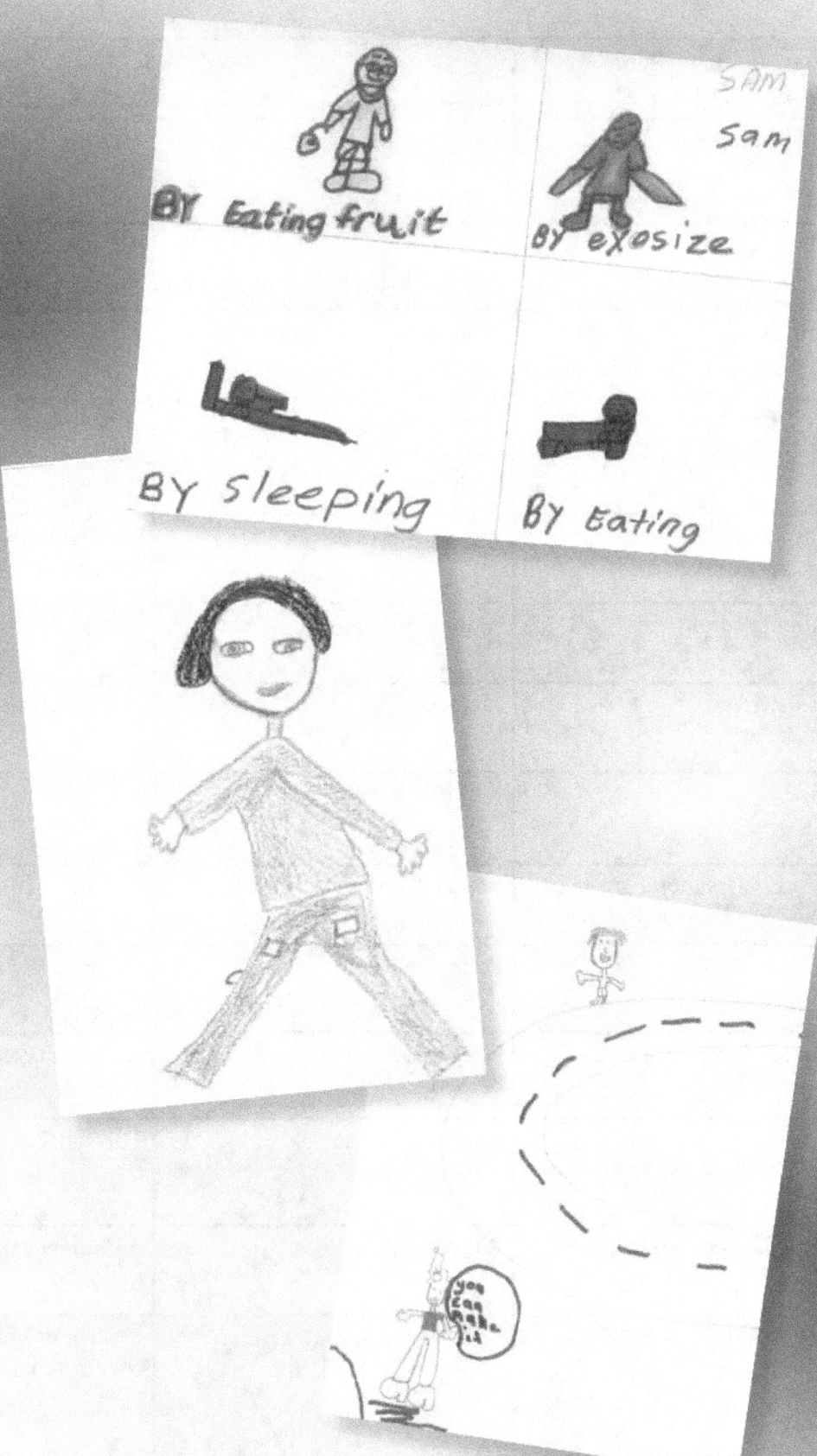

Disease	Caused by	Spread by
Chickenpox	Varicella Zoster virus	Air, direct contact
Diphtheria	*Corynebacterium diphtheriae* bacteria	Air, direct contact
Hib Disease	*Haemophilus influenzae* type b bacteria	Air, direct contact
Hepatitis A	Hepatitis A virus	Personal contact. Contaminated food or water.
Hepatitis B	Hepatitis B virus	Contact with blood or body fluids
Influenza (Flu)	Influenza virus	Air, direct contact
Measles	Measles virus	Air, direct contact
Mumps	Mumps virus	Air, direct contact
Pertussis (whooping cough)	*Bordetella pertussis* bacteria	Air, direct contact
Polio	Poliomyelitis virus	Through the mouth
Pneumococcal Disease	*Streptococcus pneumoniae* bacteria	Air, direct contact
Rotavirus	Rotavirus virus	Through the mouth
Rubella (German measles)	Rubella virus	Air, direct contact
Tetanus (lockjaw)	*Clostridium tetani* bacteria	Exposure through cuts in skin

Signs & Symptoms	Complications
Rash, fever	Bacterial infections, meningitis, encephalitis, pneumonia, death.
Sore throat, mild fever, membrane in throat, swollen neck	Heart failure, paralysis, pneumonia, death.
May be no symptoms unless bacteria enter blood.	Meningitis, epiglotittis, pneumonia, arthritis, death.
Fever, stomach pain, loss of appetite, fatigue, vomiting, jaundice, dark urine.	Liver failure, death.
Fever, headache, malaise, vomiting, arthritis.	Chronic infection, cirrhosis, liver failure, liver cancer, death.
Fever, muscle pain, sore throat, cough.	Pneumonia, Reye syndrome, myocarditis, death.
Rash, fever, cough, runny nose, pinkeye.	Pneumonia, ear infections, encephalitis, seizures, death.
Swollen salivary glands, fever, headache, malaise, muscle pain.	Meningitis, encephalitis, inflammation of testicles or ovaries, deafness.
Severe cough, runny nose, fever.	Pneumonia, seizures, brain disorders, ear infection, death.
May be no symptoms, sore throat, fever, nausea.	Paralysis, death.
Pneumonia (fever, chills, cough, chest pain).	Bacteremia (blood infection), meningitis, death.
Diarrhea, fever, vomiting	Severe diarrhea, dehydration, electrolyte imbalance, kidney and liver disease, death
Rash, fever, lymphadenopathy, malaise.	Encephalitis, arthritis/arthralgia, hemorrhage, orchitis.
Stiffness in neck, difficulty swallowing, rigid abdominal muscles, muscle spasms, fever, sweating, elevated blood pressure.	Broken bones, breathing difficulty, death.

GLOSSARY

Adverse Event — This term is used to describe a medical problem that occurs after a vaccination, which may or may not have been caused by the vaccine. (Saying adverse reaction, on the other hand, assumes that the vaccine was the cause.)

Antibody — A protein produced by the immune system that helps identify and destroy foreign substances that enter the body.

Antigen — A disease germ – generally a bacterium or virus.

Bacteremia — Presence of bacteria in the blood.

Clinical Trials — Testing of vaccines before they are licensed, during which they are given to increasingly larger groups of volunteer subjects to evaluate their safety and effectiveness.

Communicable Disease — A disease that can spread from one person to another.

Convulsion — See seizure.

Encephalitis — Inflammation of the brain.

Encephalopathy — Any illness affecting the brain.

Epidemic — A large outbreak of disease (see outbreak). A worldwide epidemic is called a pandemic.

Exposure — Contact with germs that cause disease. A person must be both exposed and susceptible to a disease to get sick from it.

Febrile Seizure — A seizure caused by a high fever.

Herd Immunity — Protection from disease in a community, due to a large enough proportion of the population having immunity to prevent the disease from spreading from person to person.

Immunity — Protection from disease. Having antibodies to a disease organism usually gives a person immunity.

Iron Lung — A cylindrical steel chamber that "breathes" for a person whose muscles that control breathing have been paralyzed. Some patients have been confined to an iron lung for life.

Local Reaction — A reaction that is confined to a small area. With vaccines, a local reaction usually refers to redness, soreness or swelling where an injection was given. A reaction that affects the body as a whole, such as a fever or bacteremia, is called a systemic reaction.

Meningitis — Inflammation of the covering of the brain or spinal cord.

Outbreak — An unusually large number of cases of a disease occurring at the same time and place, involving people who all got the disease from the same source or from each other.

Paralysis — Inability to move the muscles. Paralysis usually occurs in the arms or legs, but any muscle can become paralyzed, including those that control breathing.

Schedule — (Or vaccination schedule). The ages and/or intervals at which vaccines are recommended.

Seizure — A spell during which muscles may jerk uncontrollably, or a person stares at nothing. Usually a seizure lasts only a brief time and doesn't cause permanent harm. A seizure can have many causes, including epilepsy or other brain disorders, or a high fever (see febrile seizure). Also called convulsion or fit.

Susceptible — Vulnerable to disease. Someone who has never had a disease or been vaccinated against it is susceptible to that disease. Opposite of immune.

Toxin — Poison.

Vaccine-Preventable Disease — Any disease for which there is a vaccine.

LEARN MORE

Books

- *What Every Parent Should Know About Vaccines* by Paul A. Offit, MD and Louis M. Bell, MD. A good introduction to immunization. Includes chapters about foreign travel, how vaccines work and how they are made, and safety.

- *Vaccinating Your Child: Questions & Answers for the Concerned Parent* by Sharon G. Humiston, MD and Cynthia Goode. Another good introduction, which answers many of the questions parents have about childhood vaccinations.

- *Autism's False Prophets: Bad Science, Risky Medicine, and the Search for a Cure* by Paul A. Offit, MD. A comprehensive account of the controversy surrounding vaccines and autism.

- *Vaccine-Preventable Disease: The Forgotten Story* by Rachel M. Cunningham, Julie A. Boom, MD, and Carol J. Baker, MD. "Behind each person who has contracted a vaccine-preventable disease is the story of a life interrupted, of a family devastated. [This booklet] profiles families who have suffered the true cost of not vaccinating." Samples and ordering information can be found on the Texas Children's Hospital website at **http://www.texaschildrens.org/ carecenters/vaccine/Vaccine_Book/default.aspx**

- *Vaccines: 5th Edition*, edited by Stanley A. Plotkin, MD, Walter A. Orenstein, MD, and Paul A Offit, MD. This is a large (1,725 pages), expensive, and technically dense book. But it probably contains more information about vaccines and vaccine-preventable diseases than any other single source in the world, written by some of the world's leading experts in their field, and referencing thousands of scientific papers.

- *Epidemiology & Prevention of Vaccine-Preventable Diseases (The "Pink Book")*, edited by William L. Atkinson, MD, et al. This CDC publication is a comprehensive introduction to the principles of
vaccination, vaccines and vaccine-preventable diseases, and recommendations for vaccine use in the United States. Written for healthcare providers, it also contains information of interest to parents. Available online, or may be purchased through the Public Health Foundation (see **www.cdc.gov/vaccines/pubs/pinkbook**).

Internet

You can find vast amounts of information about vaccinations on the internet. The problem is that, unlike with book publishing, there are few controls on internet materials. Anyone can create a website or blog and say anything they want to say without having to back it up. So the question becomes: How do you know what to believe?

Of course there is no sure way to know whether information on a website is accurate or not, but several websites offer suggestions for evaluating web content. These sites include:

http://www.lib.berkeley.edu/TeachingLib/Guides/Internet/Evaluate.html

http://www.library.jhu.edu/evaluatinginformation/

http://www.nlm.nih.gov/medlineplus/webeval/webeval.html

http://www.virtualchase.com/quality/

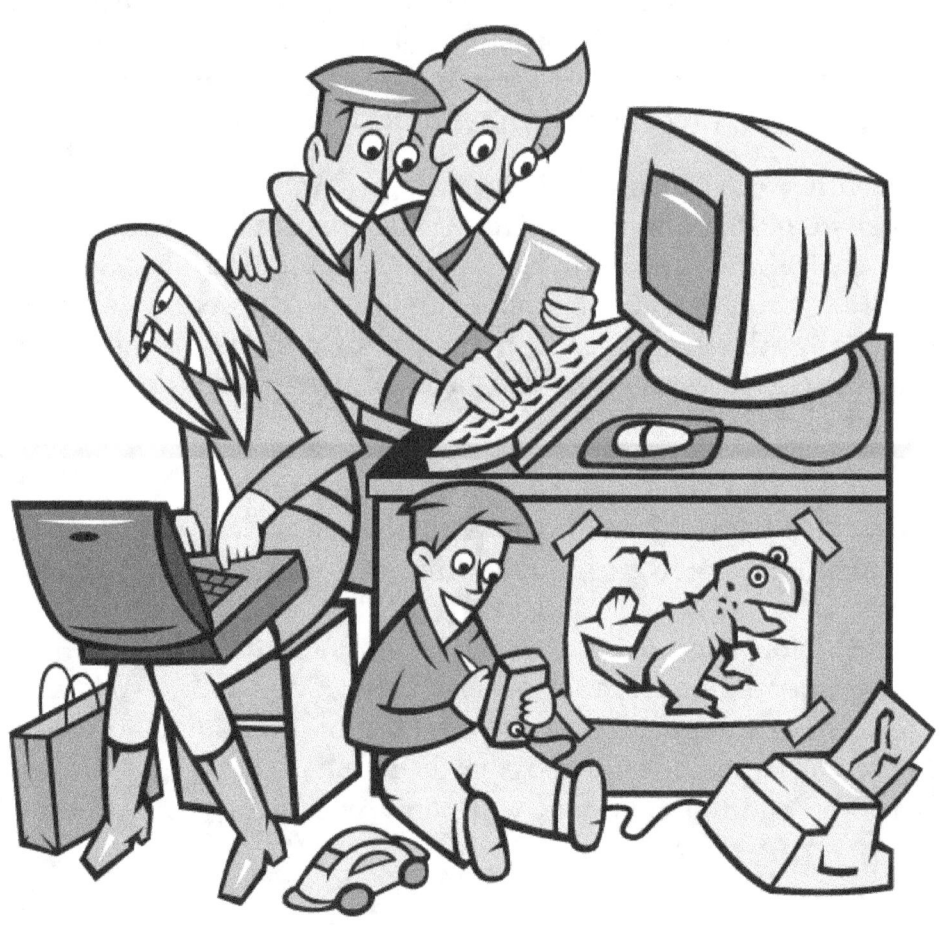

Based on information from these sources, here are a few questions to ask when trying to determine the accuracy of information you find on the web:

- Is the website's "domain" (government, education, commercial, nonprofit, etc.) appropriate for the type of information you are seeking?

- Can you identify an author or authors for the website's content?

- What are the author's credentials? Are they appropriate?

- Where did the author get his or her information? How reputable are their sources?

- If information is reproduced from other sources, does it seem to be complete, or is it edited or taken out of context? Are there links to the original source?

- What are the apparent motives of the creators of the website? To inform you? Sell you something? Influence your opinion? Make you angry?

- Can information on the website be verified?

- Does information on the website seem objective? Do there appear to be political, ideological, or other biases? Is personal opinion presented as fact?

- What is the author's tone? Is it reasonable? Uncomfortably opinionated? Ranting? Does the language seem objective, or overly biased or manipulative? Do the author's arguments rest on conspiracy theories?

- If they link to other websites, what kind of sites are they?

- Are grammar and spelling reasonably correct?

Here are some websites we like, and think you will find useful:

• CDC Websites:

  - General vaccine information: **www.cdc.gov/vaccines**

  - Information about hepatitis: **www.cdc.gov**

  - Information about flu: **www.cdc.gov/flu**

  - International travel information: **wwwn.cdc.gov/travel**

• American Academy of Pediatrics: **www.aap/org/new/immpublix.htm**

  - Information about vaccine contents: **http://www.aap.org/immunization/families/faq/Vaccineingredients.pdf**

  - Information about the vaccine schedule: **http://www.aap.org/immunization/families/faq/Vaccineschedule.pdf**

  - Information about vaccine safety: **http://www.aap.org/immunization/families/VaccineSafety_parenthandout.pdf**

• World Health Organization: **www.who.int/vaccines**

• Vaccine Education Center at the Children's Hospital of Philadelphia: **www.chop.edu/service/vaccine-education-center/home.html**

• National Network for Immunization Information: **www.immunizationinfo.org**

• Pediatrician Dr. Ari Brown's website, baby411: **www.baby411.com** (for a good piece specifically on vaccinations, see **www.windsorpeak.com/baby411/Vaccine.pdf**)

• The Autism Science Foundation: **www.autismsciencefoundation.org**

• Dr. Reddy's Pediatric Office on the Web: **www.drreddy.com/shots**

- National Vaccine Injury Compensation Program: **www.hrsa.gov/vaccinecompensation**

- Vaccine Adverse Event Reporting System: **www.vaers.hhs.gov**

- The Immunization Action Coalition's website (**www.immunize. org**) is primarily for healthcare providers, but an area of the site called "Unprotected People reports" (**www.immunize.org/ reports**/) contains reports about people who suffered injury or even death from diseases that could have been prevented by vaccines.

Telephone

- **Your state health department's immunization program.** Link to your state's immunization website from www.immuniza-tion.org/states. (Thanks to the Immunization Action Coalition for maintaining this list.)

- **CDC-INFO.** Live professionals are available 8:00 a.m. to 8:00 p.m., Monday through Friday to answer your questions about vaccines and vaccine-preventable diseases. Call 800-232-4636 (800-CDC-INFO).

Acknowledgments

The following are thanked for submitting their drawings for use in this publication:

Adriana Toungette, Alejandro Macias, Alex Cordon, Amber Blakely, Andwon Tyson, Brandon Rosillo, Cynthia Reys, Daniel Orta, Dioner Gala, Estefany, Evn Marilyn Benson, Gihasel Kahn, Henock, Iyana Williams, Jocelyn Kopfman, Jonathan Moore, Kyle Smith, Maggie Desantos, Manuela Rahimic, Marisol Baughman, Melissa Lopez, Moises, Nataly Leal, Nataneal Nistor, Ramon Perez, Riley Wright, Sam Toungette, Trent L., Vincent, Gabrielle Kroger, Rylie Jacobs, and Rachel Kroger

Department of Health and Human Services
Centers for Disease Control and Prevention
National Center for Immunization and Respiratory Disease

Live professionals are available 24 hours a day to answer your
questions about vaccines and vaccine-preventable diseases.
Call 800-232-4636 (800-CDC-INFO).

www.ingramcontent.com/pod-product-compliance
Lightning Source LLC
Chambersburg PA
CBHW081855170526
45167CB00007B/3022